JAMES L. DICKERSON has written twenty-five nonfiction books and more than two thousand magazine and newspaper articles for publications such as *Good Housekeeping, Omni, Glamour, Book-Page,* and others. An award-winning writer, he has extensive experience as a magazine and newspaper editor, book critic, and reporter. He has worked as a ~~~~~~~~~~~~~~~ including ~~~~~~~~~~~ *Times,* and ~~~~~~~~~~ he Sartoris ~~~~~~~ ist, he was ~~~~~~~~~ s involved ~~~~~~~~~ ts. In that ~~~~~~~~~ o adoptive and foster homes. He is the coauthor of *The Basics of Adoption* and the award-winning *Mojo Triangle.* He was diagnosed with autoimmune hepatitis in 2005. A graduate of the University of Mississippi, he lives in Jackson, Mississippi.

THE FIRST YEAR®

Cirrhosis

An Essential Guide for the Newly Diagnosed

James L. Dickerson

Foreword by Fredric Regenstein, MD

MARLOWE & COMPANY ■ NEW YORK

THE FIRST YEAR®—CIRRHOSIS:
An Essential Guide for the Newly Diagnosed

Published by
Marlowe & Company
An Imprint of Avalon Publishing Group, Incorporated
245 West 17th Street, 11th floor
New York, NY 10011

AVALON
publishing group incorporated

The First Year® and A Patient-Expert Walks You Through
Everything You Need to Learn and Do® are trademarks of
the Avalon Publishing Group, Inc.

Library of Congress Cataloging-in-Publication data is available.

ISBN-10: 1-56924-283-6
ISBN-13: 978-1-56924-283-4

9 8 7 6 5 4 3 2 1

Designed by Pauline Neuwirth,
  Neuwirth and Associates, Inc.

Printed in the United States of America

To my son,
Jonathan Dickerson

Contents

FOREWORD BY FREDRIC REGENSTEIN, MD   xi

ARE YOU AT RISK FOR CIRRHOSIS?   xv

INTRODUCTION   xvii

DAY 1
  Living: You Have Cirrhosis. Now What?   1
  Learning: Your Liver Is Your Best Friend   5

DAY 2
  Living: First Things First   10
  Learning: How Your Liver Works   15

DAY 3
  Living: Finding the Right Doctors   20
  Learning: Understanding the Medical Tests You Will Be Given 26

DAY 4
  Living: How Did I Get This Disease?   32
  Learning: Breaking the News to Loved Ones   35

Day 5
Living: What Should I Be Eating?   42
Learning: What You Need to Know about Hepatitis   47

Day 6
Living: Taking Your Vitamins   55
Learning: Your Disease May Be
    Caused by Drug Reactions   62

Day 7
Living: Taking Care of You   67
Learning: Autoimmune Hepatitis   71

First-Week Milestone   76

Week 2
Living: Undergoing a Liver Biopsy   77
Learning: Interpreting Your Test Results   81

Week 3
Living: Dealing with Addictions   90
Learning: Alcoholic Liver Disease   96

Week 4
Living: Building a Support Network   100
Learning: Insurance and Financial Planning   106

First-Month Milestone   114

Month 2
Living: Finding a Therapist   115
Learning: What Are My Treatment Options?   119

Month 3
Living: How Much Should I Exercise?   129
Learning: Obesity and Cirrhosis   134

Month 4
Living: What Are the Complications of Cirrhosis?   139
Learning: Coping with Complications
    When They Arise   146

Month 5
Living: Dealing with Depression   152
Learning: What Does Sleep Have to Do with It?   157

Month 6
Living: What If I Get Liver Cancer? 161
Learning: Children with Cirrhosis 168

Half-Year Milestone 173

Month 7
Living: Seniors with Cirrhosis 175
Learning: Dealing with Your Employer 181

Month 8
Living: The Healing Power of Love and Prayer 186
Learning: Alternative Treatments 193

Month 9
Living: What You Need to Know about Sex 200
Learning: Becoming a Partner in Your Care:
Conversation with an Expert—Dr. Charles Hall,
Gastroenterologist 207

Month 10
Living: Finding Information and Support
on the Internet 211
Learning: Improving Your Odds:
Conversation with an Expert—Dr. Fredric Regenstein,
Hepatologist 218

Month 11
Living: When Treatment Fails: Finding a
Transplant Center 223
Learning: If You Have to Have a Transplant 229

Month 12
Living: You Always Have Choices 236
Learning: Winning Your Battle with Cirrhosis 240

Glossary 245

Resources 249

Acknowledgments 252

Index 253

Foreword

by Fredric Regenstein, MD

FOR THE patient newly diagnosed with cirrhosis, questions abound and anxiety runs high. How much of my liver is working? What does this mean for me? How much longer do I have? Can you cut out just the bad part of my liver? Do I need to get on a transplant list? Patients with cirrhosis seeing me for the first time frequently ask these and other questions. James L. Dickerson had similar questions and he relates his personal experience in this enlightening book.

Cirrhosis is a term often misused and misunderstood by both laypersons and physicians. Cirrhosis occurs through a progressive process known as fibrosis. Over a period of many years, even decades, the fibrosis progresses through stages, culminating in the last stage of fibrosis, known as cirrhosis. Fibrosis is essentially scar tissue. The fibrosis, or scar tissue, accumulates as the liver attempts to repair itself.

Whenever the liver is injured or damaged, a sequence of events is triggered that includes the formation of scar tissue. Strictly speaking, cirrhosis can only be diagnosed with a liver biopsy. The pathologist examining the liver biopsy looks for evidence of fibrosis-forming nodules surrounding groups of liver cells. When a biopsy contains one or more complete nodules of scar tissue, cirrhosis can be diagnosed. The diagnosis of cirrhosis is not based on any specific symptom, laboratory test, X-ray, or liver scan result.

Once cirrhosis occurs, it has a number of consequences. These consequences, or cirrhotic complications, lead to abnormalities that may be detectable upon physical examination, laboratory testing, or liver scanning. Thus, when a patient presents with any number of different abnormalities, despite not having had a biopsy, cirrhosis may be presumed to be present.

Cirrhosis involves the entire liver. It does not affect just one part of the liver; therefore, it cannot be removed surgically. In the early stages of cirrhosis, laboratory tests and physical examinations may be completely normal. Patients whose tests are normal and who look "too good" to have a potentially serious problem like cirrhosis have fooled and surprised many physicians.

Unlike virtually all other organs in the body, the liver receives most of its blood supply from a vein, rather than an artery. The main vein supplying blood to the liver is the portal vein. The portal vein contains virtually all of the blood draining from the spleen and intestines. This peculiarity of the liver circulation allows the liver to interact with, process, modify, and store the food, chemicals, vitamins, medications, and toxins absorbed across the gastrointestinal tract. This unique circulation is responsible for many of the symptoms and complications that occur as the cirrhosis progresses. These are well reviewed and described in this book (Month 4).

As scar tissue and cirrhotic nodules form in the liver, blood vessels are compressed. The more the cirrhosis progresses, the more the blood vessels become compressed, making it difficult for blood to flow through the liver. As blood flowing through the portal vein meets resistance in the liver, the blood begins to back up, the same way traffic does when there is a lane closure on the freeway. Like the traveler stuck in traffic, looking for a shortcut around the freeway tie-up, blood flowing to the cirrhotic liver searches for an alternate route back to the heart. Many times the alternate route involves small veins in the stomach and esophagus. Over time, these veins may enlarge and become varicose veins (varices). As these veins were not designed to carry large amounts of blood, they can sometime rupture, leading to one of the most dreaded complications of cirrhosis, bleeding varices.

Hepatic encephalopathy is another disabling complication of cirrhosis (see Month 4). In normal individuals, toxin-filled blood coming from the intestines must first pass through the liver, where it is purified, before getting back to the heart. In patients with cirrhosis, some of the toxin-filled blood bypasses the liver by traveling through the newly formed varices around the stomach, esophagus, and elsewhere. Once these poisons get to the heart, they are pumped to the rest of the body.

When toxin-filled blood arrives at the brain, it causes hepatic encephalopathy. Patients with encephalopathy may not be able to drive or function at work. People with advanced cirrhosis and severe encephalopathy may lapse into a coma with little or no warning. Sometimes the coma may be caused by medications prescribed by their physicians for relief of pain, anxiety, depression, or sleep disorders. Certain toxins make the brain more sensitive to the effects of these medications. In addition, medications taken by mouth may reach blood levels two or three times higher than in a normal person, due to blood bypassing the liver. This is a major reason why so many medications contain cautions or warnings about use in patients with liver disease.

Another organ affected by blood not being able to flow through the liver is the spleen. When blood backs up into the spleen, the spleen increases in size (this is called splenomegaly). Physicians examining patients with liver disorders always look for signs of an enlarged spleen, one of the few findings present on physical examination in the early stages of cirrhosis. An enlarged spleen traps white blood cells and platelets, leading to low levels of white blood cells (WBC count) and platelets (platelet count). A depressed platelet count is one of the most frequent laboratory abnormalities in patients with cirrhosis (see Day 3). Removal of the spleen is occasionally recommended for patients with cirrhosis and extremely low platelet counts; however, the procedure is much more dangerous in patients with cirrhosis and should be avoided if possible.

Because the liver has many different functions and because many of the complications of cirrhosis occur as a result of changes in the way blood flows through and around the liver, it is very hard to answer one of the questions most often asked by patients: "How much of my liver is working?" Unlike with the heart or the kidney, where your doctor can tell you the exact percentage the heart is pumping or the kidney filtering, there is no similar measure of liver function. Liver specialists must look at a variety of different tests and symptoms in order to assess how far along a patient may be in the course of their disease. Even the most experienced specialists cannot accurately say what percentage of the liver is functioning.

People may have cirrhosis for many years before they or their physicians become aware of any problem. In the early stages, patients are labeled as having "compensated cirrhosis." Patients with compensated cirrhosis have an excellent prognosis. Things begin to change once a person develops one of the serious complications (ascites, encephalopathy, bleeding varices) of cirrhosis. Development of these complications is referred to as decompensation. Once a patient develops decompensation, the prognosis becomes guarded. Without liver transplantation, approximately half the patients with decompensation will die within five years. Once a person develops signs or symptoms of decompensation, they should ask their doctor to refer them to a specialist, preferably one affiliated with a liver transplant center.

Cirrhosis used to be thought of as a "dead end": once scar tissue was put down in the liver, it was there for the rest of your life. We now understand that the process by which scar tissue (fibrosis) is formed is a dynamic process, or a "two-way street." If you treat, or better yet cure, the underlying cause of the cirrhosis, the scar tissue may go away. Thus, in some patients with cirrhosis caused by hepatitis B or hepatitis C, treatment of their hepatitis leads to the disappearance of their cirrhosis. There appears to be a "point of no return" where the cirrhosis is so advanced the liver will never return to normal; however, treatment of the underlying condition may lead to stabilization, such that there is little, if any, worsening in the cirrhosis for the remainder of a person's life.

In this book, James L. Dickerson has provided you with a road map for how to navigate your way through the confusion and fear that results once you have been diagnosed with cirrhosis. He offers important insights gained from his own research, experience, and anxiety. This book will be a useful resource as you learn more about your unique situation. You will find the information provided in this book extremely helpful when you interact with your physicians, perform independent research, and establish your own individual way of coping and living with this condition.

—Dr. Fredric Regenstein *is chief of clinical hepatology at the Tulane University Center for Abdominal Transplant in New Orleans. He has authored and coauthored numerous articles on the subjects of viral hepatitis and liver transplantation. His current areas of interest are prevention of recurrent hepatitis in transplant patients and management of late complications in liver transplant recipients.*

Are you at risk for cirrhosis?

> *My uncle has cirrhosis and I'm afraid*
> *I might have it, too. I wish there was*
> *a home test I could take before I see a doctor.*
>
> —TEMEKA J.

There are no blood or urine tests you can take at home to determine if you have cirrhosis, but there is a symptom questionnaire you can take that will let you know if you have enough symptoms to be of concern.

If you answer yes to any five of the following questions, you should make an appointment with your doctor to discuss your symptoms. A score of five or higher *does not mean* that you have cirrhosis. It does indicate that your body is undergoing changes that are consistent with numerous diseases, including cirrhosis.

○ Do people often tell you that you have bad breath?
○ Are your palms often red for no apparent reason?
○ Do you have spiderlike blood vessels that are visible on your chest?
○ Do you have frequent indigestion?
○ Have you ever been diagnosed with hepatitis B or C?
○ Have you ever had unprotected sex with anyone who has hepatitis B or C?
○ Do you drink more than one alcoholic beverage a day?
○ Are your stools ever light-clay colored?
○ Within the past month, has your urine been dark yellow or brown?
○ Do you have a tattoo or body piercing?
○ Have you ever had oral-anal sex?
○ Are your ankles ever swollen for no apparent reason?
○ Do you ever experience severe itching?
○ If female, are your breasts shrinking?
○ If female, has your menstrual cycle recently changed?
○ Do you find it more difficult to remember recent events?
○ Do you have lupus or rheumatoid arthritis?
○ Do you often have reactions to prescription drugs?
○ If male, have you noticed a loss of interest in sex?
○ Have you ever taken an antibiotic that made your joints ache?

- Have you recently eaten raw oysters or undercooked shrimp?
- Are you experiencing hair loss?
- Has your skin come in contact with pesticides or other toxic chemicals?
- Has the normal pink color of your fingernail bed turned white, causing the half-moon circles at the base of the nail to disappear?
- Do you have hemorrhoids?
- If female, have you noticed increased underarm hair?

IN A SENTENCE:

> *Early diagnosis of cirrhosis depends on the patient's ability to recognize important changes taking place in his or her body.*

Introduction

IF YOU are reading this book, the odds are that you or someone you know has cirrhosis. If so, you have already received the bad news. The good news is yet to come: cirrhosis is not a death sentence—and you have every reason to be hopeful.

You should know that you are not alone. More than twenty-five million Americans are afflicted with liver and gallbladder disease, which translates to nearly 400,000 new cases of chronic liver disease or cirrhosis annually. For a disease that plays such a prominent role in our lives, you would think cirrhosis would have more public visibility than it does. You seldom see charity events or telethons or celebrity endorsements in support of cirrhosis research, as you do with other diseases. That is unfortunate, because ignorance about liver disease increases the odds of getting it—and of suffering unnecessary complications from it.

Cirrhosis is a degenerative disease in which normal liver cells become damaged and then are replaced by scar tissue. The most common causes of cirrhosis are excessive alcohol consumption, hepatitis, autoimmune disease, and complications from prescription and over-the-counter drugs. The less common causes of cirrhosis are inherited diseases such as:

O Wilson's disease, a disorder characterized by accumulations of copper in the liver, brain, kidneys, and corneas
O A lack of alpha 1-antitrypsin, a liver enzyme
O The absence of a milk-digesting enzyme called galactosemia
O Glycogen storage disease, an inability to convert sugar to energy
O Hemochromatosis, an absorption deficit in which excess iron is deposited in the liver, pancreas, heart, and other organs

Cirrhosis is often termed a "silent killer" because it shows no symptoms in its early stages. It can take years to develop, sometimes thirty years or more, or it can develop very quickly and run its course in a relatively short period of time. Once symptoms are indicated, they are often vague—mild stomach discomfort, sleepiness, hemorrhoids, or fatigue—and often attributed to other, less serious causes, such as indigestion or anxiety. As the disease progresses, the symptoms become more alarming.

In the later stages of the disease, the whites of the eyes and the skin become yellow because of the liver's inability to process bilirubin; the urine turns dark yellow or brown; the skin itches for no apparent reason; and the patient has problems sleeping, becomes forgetful, and has problems concentrating.

Also in the later stages of the disease, the patient may neglect hygiene: perhaps he wears the same clothing day after day, when previously he put on clean clothing each day, or he may stop brushing his hair and teeth for no apparent reason. This occurs because the patient's brain is exposed to toxins that a healthy liver would normally filter out of the blood. The most common effect of increased toxins in the brain is changed behavior. Patients do things that loved ones call "out of character."

Cirrhosis is a chronic disease that causes liver failure over an extended period of time, with liver transplantation the only treatment for the disease when it is in the end stages. As with many conditions, the earlier cirrhosis is diagnosed, the better your chances for successful treatment and recovery. Fortunately, new advances in medicine have given hope to many patients with cirrhosis. Patients whose cirrhosis was caused by hepatitis B or C usually respond well to treatment, and patients with **autoimmune hepatitis** are responsive to drug therapy 80 percent of the time.

What happened to me

My interest in cirrhosis took a circuitous route. In the months before my diagnosis, I was writing a book about an ancient killer called yellow fever, an infectious viral disease that aggressively attacks the liver and digestive tract. In mild cases, the symptoms are similar to those of the flu, and are often misdiagnosed, but in serious cases, known as the toxic phase, the patient develops a high temperature and then experiences liver failure.

In the early stages, yellow fever is sometimes difficult to detect since symptoms overlap those associated with malaria, hepatitis, and poisoning of various kinds; but in its toxic phase, patients develop **jaundice** and vomit blood.

During the period when I was reading autopsy reports for yellow fever victims, I developed mild stomach distress, the sort of indigestion that we have all experienced from time to time. I didn't think anything of it at first, but when it persisted beyond a week, I went to see a physician, Dr. Kim Ellis. She said my stomach distress could be caused by any number of things, but was probably due to gastritis. She gave me prescriptions for an antibiotic named **Cipro** and a heartburn medication named Nexium.

Neither medicine immediately improved my condition, but since my discomfort was minor to begin with, I wasn't concerned. However, toward the end of the first week of medication, I noticed a new set of symptoms. My knee joints began to ache. My urine was darker than usual. And I began to itch for no apparent reason. I rationalized those symptoms. I told myself they were due to drinking insufficient amounts of water, lack of exercise, or an allergic reaction to something I didn't know I was allergic to.

About a week later, a friend stopped by to visit and gave me a quizzical look. "When's the last time you looked in the mirror?" she asked.

"This morning, I guess—when I shaved."

"You didn't notice anything unusual?"

"No, not really."

She leaned in closer to my face. "Hmmmm," she said. "You should look again. Your eyes are yellow."

I don't have to tell you, considering the project I was working on, what hearing those words did to me. I rushed to a mirror and saw for myself that my eyes were indeed yellow. "Yellow fever," I sighed, fearing the obvious. "I've got yellow fever."

Later that day, I returned to the doctor who had prescribed medication for my "gastritis." Dr. Ellis ordered a urinalysis and a blood test to evaluate my **liver enzymes**. When the results showed that I was experiencing liver failure, she quickly referred me to a gastroenterologist, who saw me two days later. This gastroenterologist, who shall be nameless, examined my blood work, poked around my stomach a bit, and then promptly left the examining room to dictate his notes into a recorder located just outside the door. The entire examination took less than five minutes.

The doctor's voice reminded me of a sports play-by-play announcer: it was so loud that it surely carried into the busy street outside the building. I really didn't want to overhear his diagnosis from the other side of a closed door, so I stuck my fingers into my ears and paced about the room, looking at the anatomical charts on the walls.

When the doctor returned to the examining room, he asked me to sit down so that he could discuss my condition. Speaking gravely, but avoiding eye contact, he pointed to a chart that showed the liver and gallbladder, and said: "Your problems may be caused by your gallbladder, but my concern is that you have cancer that probably originated in your colon and spread to your liver and pancreas. Let's do a CT scan tomorrow."

I was devastated. I don't really remember much that happened over the next few hours. Time seemed to stop. The next morning I was up at daybreak, after fasting since midnight. The technician who performed the CT scan finished by 10 AM and told me that the results had already been faxed to my doctor. Already faxed? Was that good news or bad news? I went home to wait for a call from my doctor. He didn't call that day—or the next. I suffered through the weekend, certain that he would call first thing Monday morning. Why wouldn't he? He received the test results on Thursday. I called and left a message for him to please give me a call. He ignored me. For a full week I sweated out the results of that test.

Meanwhile, I found out everything I could about liver disease on the Internet. The first thing that jumped out at me was that if you had liver, pancreatic, and colon cancer, all combined, you would be lucky to live six weeks. Why, I wondered, would my doctor eat up such a big hunk of my life expectancy by not calling me? Was the news so bad that he didn't have the heart to tell me?

Finally, I heard from the doctor's office. Exactly ten days after the CT scan was done and the results sent to my doctor, his nurse called to tell me that the scan had uncovered no abnormalities. I was speechless. However, she continued: "We want you to come in tomorrow for an ultrasound scan."

The ultrasound scan was not too bad as medical procedures go, just a lot of sticky gel smeared on my stomach and chest; before I left the office, I pleaded with the technician to give me the results. She agreed to do that after giving the images to the radiologist for interpretation. She disappeared for a few minutes. When she returned, she told me that the ultrasound had found no abnormalities.

I went home to wait for the "official" test results from my doctor. Of course, I heard nothing. One week later I received a note in the mail that informed me that the test had found no abnormalities. The note also said, "Please come into the office tomorrow so that we can discuss your condition."

I declined the invitation. Instead, I returned to Dr. Ellis and asked her to find me another specialist. When I told her what had happened, her eyes welled up. "I'm so sorry," she said. She reached out and gently touched my arm, a sympathetic gesture more comforting than any prescription she could have written.

Most doctors, I suspect, have no idea how important compassionate gestures are in a time of crisis. The prospect of dying wasn't on my mind at that moment. But what bothered me was the lack of sensitivity on the part of the specialist. Didn't anyone in medical school tell him that before he suggested to patients that they had multiple cancers he should *first* run a few tests? Didn't anyone tell him that he had a responsibility to report to his patients in a timely manner on tests of a life-and-death nature?

Dr. Ellis got me an appointment with a gastroenterologist named Dr. Charles Hall, who arranged for a series of new tests: additional blood work, an ultrasound and a liver scan, a nuclear medicine test that involves the injection of radioactive particles into the bloodstream. I liked Dr. Hall right away. He asked lots of questions about my symptoms and seemed eager to get to the root of my problem. When he told me that his wife was a former newspaper reporter, I knew I was in the right office. He seemed concerned about my condition, but he didn't jump to any conclusions about the cause.

He said that my stomach problems and my high liver-enzyme test scores could be totally unrelated.

When he got the results of the ultrasound, they showed nothing significant, but my liver enzymes were still high, four or five times higher than they should have been, and the liver scan indicated that my liver was dumping some of its functions onto my spleen. "The only way to know exactly what is going on in your liver is to do a biopsy," said Dr. Hall. "You've only got one liver. We've got to do what we can to take care of it."

The biopsy itself was uneventful. They gave me a sedative, which caused me to doze off for a moment. When I awoke, the procedure was over. I felt no pain and the nurse told me that there had been no problems during the procedure. They asked me to remain in the hospital for a couple of hours for observation. They didn't tell me why, but I knew it was so that they could be certain that the needle used in the procedure had not perforated any of my other organs and caused internal bleeding.

Several days later I returned to Dr. Hall's office for the results.

"You don't have cancer," he said, pausing just long enough for me to savor that bit of good news, before he continued. "But you do have cirrhosis of the liver."

"How is that possible?" I asked. "I don't drink. I've never done drugs. Earlier tests showed that I don't have hepatitis. How could I have cirrhosis?"

"You have **cryptogenic cirrhosis**," he explained. "Only 5 to 10 percent of cases fall in that category. It's called 'crypto' because we don't know the cause."

Since I was in good health otherwise, Dr. Hall told me to start taking one-a-day vitamins, and come back to see him in three months, at which time I would be evaluated for a liver transplant (doctors do that years before they think there will be a need so they can better plan your treatment). That was it! No miracle drugs. No therapy or treatment. No road map for recovery. You've got cirrhosis—go home and take your vitamins.

Dr. Hall's one-a-day vitamin prescription is standard procedure after a cirrhosis diagnosis. A treatment plan cannot be devised until the cause of a patient's cirrhosis is determined—and that takes time. Meanwhile, regardless of the cause of the disease, it is a certainty that the liver is struggling to maintain a proper vitamin balance.

"Between now and your next visit," Dr. Hall said, "I want you to read everything you can find about cirrhosis of the liver. Some of what you will read will be encouraging. Other parts will be pretty nasty." As he was walking out of the examining room, he turned and paused a moment, his face reflecting concern. "We'll get you through this."

What I liked about Dr. Hall during those first office visits—and what I still like about him—is his ability to inspire confidence. I don't think they teach that in medical school. Wherever that quality came from in him, I believe it was the reason I never experienced depression that first year, not for one moment.

After I left his office the day of the diagnosis, I took his advice and logged on to Amazon.com, where I discovered that the only books offered about cirrhosis were written for physicians and researchers, and most of them were out of print. There are some good books on the subject of hepatitis and liver disease in general, but their focus is not on cirrhosis and they only contained a few pages of helpful information.

The more I researched cirrhosis, the more convinced I became that Cipro was the likely cause of my jaundice. If so, it was a serendipitous event that led to the discovery of my cirrhosis. Without the sudden appearance of jaundice, I would not have had a reason to undergo a liver function test—and without the test it may have been months or years before my cirrhosis would have been detected.

While I was taking my vitamins and waiting for my next visit with Dr. Hall, I was distracted from my own problems by the arrival of Hurricane Katrina. I live about 170 miles from the Gulf Coast, near Jackson, Mississippi, but I was nonetheless in the storm's path and experienced eighty-mile-an-hour winds that ripped off portions of my roof and left me in the dark for days without electricity, water, or food. The nights were long and hot, and my neighborhood was silent since almost everyone except me had fled.

There wasn't much to do, so I got caught up on my reading and spent a lot of time thinking about my disease. I never felt angry about my diagnosis. What I felt was a sense of practicality. If something happened to me, I wondered, what would become of my manuscripts and research papers?

When my next round of blood tests showed no improvement in my condition, Dr. Hall referred me to Dr. Fredric Regenstein, the chief of clinical hepatology at the Tulane University Center for Abdominal Transplant in New Orleans. Unfortunately, the center had been uprooted because of Katrina and had been temporarily relocated at a hospital in Covington, a small community north of New Orleans.

As I was waiting for confirmation of my appointment, an interesting thing happened: the gastroenterologist who had told me that he thought I had cancer that had spread from my colon to my liver called to talk to me about a letter I had written to his medical group complaining about the treatment I had received. The gastroenterologist said he was "devastated" by the letter.

"I have lived with, slept with that letter ever since I read it," he explained. "It was the most powerful letter I have ever read, positive or negative." He went on to say that he had made changes in his office procedures as a result of the letter. At the end of the conversation, he asked about my condition. I told him that I had been diagnosed with cirrhosis and was waiting for an appointment with a doctor at a liver transplant center.

"I would be happy to meet with you if you would like to discuss it further," he said. "If you have any ideas on how I can become a better doctor, I would like to hear them."

I didn't have any suggestions, beyond those contained in the letter, but I felt he was sincere in soliciting ideas from me and I appreciated the invitation. Who knows? He may yet get a list of suggestions from me. But I tell you this story to demonstrate the importance of speaking up should you ever experience problems with a physician.

A couple of weeks later, I was at Lakeview Regional Medical Center at Covington, on the northern end of Lake Pontchartrain, for my evaluation. My sister and a friend were kind enough to drive me to the hospital, a trip of about four hours. (The good company was a great diversion.) The center was larger than I expected, considering its suburban location, and I was pleasantly surprised at how spotlessly clean the walls and floors were, especially after the hurricane's muddy devastation, which I had seen on television. Once inside the hospital, I made my way to the second floor, suite 206, where the temporary offices for the transplant center were announced with scrawled handwriting on a piece of notepaper taped to a nondescript door.

I was a little apprehensive about meeting Dr. Regenstein because I knew how important it was that I like him and trust him. Meeting a new doctor under those circumstances is like meeting a blind date that your friends have arranged for you. You know almost instantly whether there will be a connection. That was certainly the case with Dr. Regenstein. Within minutes of meeting him I knew that I liked him and I was willing to trust him with my life. Another few minutes, and I felt that he was the most competent person I had ever met in any field.

Dr. Regenstein asked me lots of questions, some no doubt for the benefit of the student doctor who was intently observing the interview. Once Dr. Regenstein asked me all his questions, he asked if I had any questions. I did. I had a typewritten list that included questions such as:

- What is Tulane's mortality rate for liver transplants, and how many transplants do you do in an average year?
- What is my Child-Pugh score?
- If I don't need a transplant for five or six years, will my age be a factor in your decision to give me a transplant?
- Should I be vaccinated for hepatitis?

Dr. Regenstein laughed. "We aren't doing *any* transplants at the moment because of the storm." As far as my Child-Pugh score was concerned (and I will explain the significance of the rating scale later in the book, on page 87), he said that I was a Class A, which I later learned translated to a life expectancy of fifteen to twenty years, provided I developed no complications. He said that my age would not be a factor in five years if I needed a transplant and he advised me to be vaccinated for **hepatitis A** and **B** as soon as I returned home. It was at that point that Dr. Regenstein said something that changed my entire perspective about my disease—and gave me a thesis for this book.

"Those are all great questions," he said. "But you didn't ask the most important question."

"No," I said. "What . . . ?"

"You should have asked if there is anything I can do to treat your disease, or reverse its progress."

I was stunned. Everything I had read had painted a pretty bleak prognosis for cirrhosis. Emotionally, I had prepared myself for a transplant. Did he know something I didn't know? Of course, he did.

"Well," I asked, "is there anything you can do?"

"I don't know yet, but I do know those are the two questions you should keep asking. I would like for you to sign a release so that I can request the actual slides from your biopsy. I would like to go over them myself."

"Fine," I said. "I'm curious. Have you ever disagreed with a biopsy report?"

Dr. Regenstein grinned. "I almost always disagree."

I left Dr. Regenstein's office that day feeling very optimistic, even though nothing really had happened except for an exchange of information. On the way back home, thinking about what he had told me, I realized that following his advice about the best questions to ask was the most important thing that a cirrhosis patient could do. In other words, *recovery begins with a question.*

A couple of weeks after my visit with Dr. Regenstein, I received a call from Dr. Hall's nurse, who asked me to stop by the office. "Dr. Regenstein called me about your case," Dr. Hall said. "After looking over your biopsy slides, he thinks you have a condition called autoimmune hepatitis."

"Is that good news or is it bad news?"

"Good news," said Dr. Hall. "Autoimmune hepatitis can be treated with drugs."

Dr. Hall explained that autoimmune hepatitis was not really hepatitis, but rather a class of autoimmune diseases like **lupus**. It occurs when the body's immune system attacks specific organs as if they were invading organisms. In my case, my body attacked my liver, with cirrhosis the end result.

Dr. Hall said that he was going to place me on two drugs, a steroid named **prednisone** and an antirejection drug named **azathioprine**. He explained that 80 percent of autoimmune hepatitis patients who took the drugs went into remission.

When I returned home, I had an e-mail from Dr. Regenstein informing me of his diagnosis. "Hopefully," he wrote, "you will never need a liver transplant."

How to use this book

The one thing that all doctors seem to agree on about cirrhosis is that long-term survival depends as much on the patient as it does on the physician. In other words, the patients who have the most information about what they should and should not do to control their disease are the patients who have the best chance for a long life.

When I took Dr. Hall's advice to read everything I could about cirrhosis, I was disappointed not to find any books on the subject. There is plenty of material on the Internet, but it is difficult to weed out the bogus sites—and there are many of those—from the authoritative sites that offer safe, helpful information. Of course, with a life-threatening disease like cirrhosis, bad information is the last thing a patient needs.

I decided to write about the disease so that people like me could safely navigate through what is essentially a devastating diagnosis. I wrote *The First Year: Cirrhosis* for people like myself, individuals who have been diagnosed with a disease that they probably know nothing about. I had always heard that cirrhosis was a disease that was limited to alcoholics. That's not true. Cirrhosis can develop from several sources, many of which are unrelated to alcohol consumption. The more you read about this disease, the more you appreciate its complexity.

This book will provide you with a schedule that will help you learn what you need to know about the disease. I encourage you to adapt the information I present to you to your own needs. My goal is to guide you through the first year of living with cirrhosis, beginning with the day you are diagnosed. The first seven chapters are designed for you to read each day of the first week. The next three chapters will guide you through the second, third, and fourth weeks of the first month, and the next eleven chapters will provide a program for learning about cirrhosis and taking care of yourself during the remaining months of the first year.

I have divided each chapter into two sections, called "Living" and "Learning." The "Living" section is meant to help you with the emotional, social, and practical issues you face on a day-to-day basis, while the "Learning" section is meant to give the facts you need to manage your health. When you see a word or phrase in **boldface**, that is an indication that you can find a definition in the glossary at the end of the book.

I have tried to make the book as interactive as possible by providing you with questions to ask your health-care providers. As I pointed out earlier, I asked my own doctor a list of questions that were all very good, as far as questions go, but that were the wrong questions at that point in my treatment. I want to help you ask your doctor the right questions at the right time, because I know that your peace of mind will depend on getting the right answers.

I will not prescribe

Since I am not a medical doctor, I will not prescribe treatments or medications for you in this book. What I will do is let you know what has worked and not worked for me, what your options are in a given situation, and what experts say about various aspects of the disease. I want to provide you with as many options as I can to enable you to take charge of your disease and manage your own treatment. As a social worker, I *will* prescribe on matters related to your emotional well-being.

It is my hope that what you learn in this book will make a difference in your life. No one has all the answers you need. The patients who do the best job of managing this disease are the patients who are proactive in their choice of treatments and diets. My goal is to provide you with options, not opinions—and to answer the questions you will have after hearing your diagnosis:

- ○ What is cirrhosis and how did I get it?
- ○ How long do I have to live?
- ○ What treatment options do I have?
- ○ What can I do to stay healthy?
- ○ How is my disease likely to affect others?
- ○ Should I tell friends and family members?
- ○ What complications can I expect?
- ○ What is the worst—and the best—scenario for my disease?
- ○ What foods should I eat and what foods should I avoid?
- ○ Can I still drink beer or wine?
- ○ Does having cirrhosis increase my odds of developing liver cancer?
- ○ Will I need a liver transplant? If so, how long in advance should I prepare?

Keep on learning

Cirrhosis is a chronic illness. Even if your doctors are able to put your disease in remission, you will always have the resulting scar tissue in your liver. The question is not so much how to make it go away as it is how to live with it. By the end of your first year with the disease, you will understand that your survival and well-being is a learning process that greatly depends on your willingness to pursue new knowledge.

I encourage you to continue the learning process you began by reading this book. New discoveries are made every day. You may never know about those discoveries unless you take an activist approach and monitor newspapers, magazines, and medical Web sites for stories about the latest information in treating the disease.

IN A SENTENCE:

The first step to living with cirrhosis is to ask your doctor questions, the most important being "What can you do to treat this disease?"

living

You Have Cirrhosis.
Now What?

I just looked at the doctor, saying nothing,
because I thought he was talking to someone else,
even though there were only the two of us
in the room.

—Bobby T.

YOU HAVE probably read stories about people who have been diagnosed with life-threatening diseases. Invariably, they say that "time stopped" or they felt "stunned" or they simply sat there, "frozen" by the news.

When you found yourself in that position, it probably surprised you that you experienced all those emotions—and more. In addition to your initial reaction, you probably felt overwhelmed, perhaps even out of control. There are fancy words for all those emotions, but there is no better word to describe what you felt than *fear*. You may have noticed that your doctor didn't talk a lot after giving you the bad news. That's because he knows that the basic response to fear is flight, and all those complicated reactions you are feeling are all aspects of flight.

Of course, even though you didn't jump up out of your chair and flee, you probably did the psychological equivalent with your emotions. You withdrew into yourself. Your doctor knows that explanations would be lost on you in your current state, so he most likely did not volunteer additional information until your next visit.

Of course, he asked you if you had any questions, and he was prepared to answer them, but few patients, after receiving a bad diagnosis, have many questions, other than "Are you sure? Is it possible that you are mistaken?"

You probably didn't begin to cope with your diagnosis until you left the doctor's office. If someone accompanied you to the office, their question "What happened?" brought you back to reality because you had to actually verbalize the diagnosis.

> *When I waked in the morning, the first thought would be,* Oh, my wretched soul, what shall I do, where shall I go?
>
> —THE REVEREND HENRY ALLINE

The above thought, shared by a nineteenth-century minister in a biography published in 1806, was not inspired by a life-threatening diagnosis, but rather by what the author called a religious "melancholy." However, the sentiment is identical to what many people feel upon being told that they have a disease that might cut their life short.

Exhaustion is usually the first response your body has to your new awareness of your own mortality. Not the kind of exhaustion you get from jogging around the block a few times. Rather, it is the kind of exhaustion that seems to come from someplace deep inside yourself, a place you never knew existed. Not until the next morning, when you see the sunlight creeping in your window, seemingly with a new sense of urgency, will you really begin to come to terms with your diagnosis.

Most people go through the same feelings that accompany the loss of a loved one:

- ○ Fear: "Something is trying to kill me."
- ○ Sadness: "I have nothing to look forward to."
- ○ Guilt: "I must be sick because of something that I have done."
- ○ Confusion: "What am I supposed to do next?"

You won't go through all those emotions on the first day. The process may be drawn out over several weeks or months. Some people stay in one emotion, spinning their wheels like a car on ice. Others go through them like a checklist. The final emotion is a sense of relief that follows satisfactory answers to the final question, "What am I supposed to do next?" Once that emotional gauntlet has been navigated, you may go through some or all of the five stages of grief:

- Denial and isolation
- Anger
- Bargaining
- Depression
- Acceptance

When faced with a serious diagnosis, there are, at times, no words to describe how you feel. It may surprise you that the people who love you the most may have the most difficulty understanding your pain. That's because love and support, though invaluable, are not a substitute for experience in situations like this. If your loved ones have never experienced what you are going through, they have nothing to fall back on to help them empathize with you. They will say all the right words, but these may ring hollow. You may find it easier to connect with a stranger who has gone through the same experience than with your loving spouse or parents.

One result of that failed connection is a sense of isolation. For the first time in your life, you realize that facing a life-threatening illness is something that you truly must experience alone. Once you understand that, you may go through another stage—anger. The target of your anger will likely have nothing to do with your illness. You might direct your anger at anything that moves—at your loved ones for making you feel isolated; at your doctor for giving you the bad news; at the disease for choosing you when it had so many others to consider; at your parents for bringing you into the world; at your siblings for being the lucky ones; and the list goes on and on.

Luckily, the anger you feel will be of short duration, primarily because it will soon become apparent to you that your anger makes no sense and is not helping you fight your disease. At that point, you may try to bargain your way out of your difficulty. If you are religious, you will bargain with God and promise to do wonderful things for the world, if only you can be spared from this disease. If you are not religious, you may bargain with yourself in the belief that good works will overshadow the disease.

Bargaining gives you a sense of accomplishment while you are doing it, but there will come a time when you realize that it is futile. That old saying, "If it sounds too good to be true, it probably is" may apply to your bargaining efforts with God. If it was true that you could bargain your way out of a life-threatening illness, then everyone would do it and we would all live forever. After realizing that bargaining isn't the answer to your problem, you may feel a sense of depression unlike anything you have ever experienced. If you are lucky, the next stage—depression—will be of short duration. If it persists beyond several weeks, you may want to seek professional help to get you over the hump and into the final stage—acceptance.

The most important thing for you to do at this stage is to concentrate on the present. There will be time later to ponder the past, just as there will be time to plan for the future. Accept your situation for what it is. Look around you. Almost everyone has something wrong with their life. Many people have diseases much worse than cirrhosis. Stay focused on what you have to do to feel better. Your life may depend on it.

IN A SENTENCE:

It is all right to be afraid at first—know that you will find the strength to take control of your health.

learning

Your Liver Is Your Best Friend

EVERYONE KNOWS they have a liver, but few people know where it is located: it is in the right upper quadrant of the abdomen and extends slightly below the rib cage (you can feel it with your fingertips if you take a deep breath). Nor do many understand its importance: it is the one organ whose sole purpose is to protect you against disease and to keep you alive. Unlike the heart, whose main purpose is to circulate blood throughout your body, or your lungs, whose main purpose is to gather oxygen, the liver performs over one hundred complicated functions, each of them essential for your survival.

Think of your liver as a refinery. It cleanses the body of toxic substances. It manufactures and sends to other organs chemicals that are needed to function properly. It converts fats, proteins, and carbohydrates into chemicals necessary for growth and development. It stores extra vitamins, minerals, and sugars until they are needed. It **metabolizes** alcohol. It synthesizes chemicals that are essential in blood clotting. It controls the production and excretion of cholesterol. It controls hormone balance. And it processes drugs that are needed to treat disease elsewhere in the body.

Every minute, about one-quarter of your blood supply passes through your liver. Most of that blood is carried by the **portal vein**, which travels from the intestines—where the blood gathers nutrients—and then to the liver; and by the **hepatic artery**, which takes oxygenated blood from the aorta to the liver, where it is dispersed by capillaries called **sinusoids**. Since the liver has a dual blood supply, it is less susceptible to being shut down by a single clot, as can happen with the heart and other organs (one measure of the value that nature has put on the liver).

There are many chemicals associated with liver function, but two of the most important are **albumin** and **bilirubin**. Albumin is the major protein present in the blood. It is essential for the proper maintenance of fluid balances in the body. Decreased albumin production is associated with increased fluid levels in the body. Bilirubin is a chemical compound that is produced in the body when red blood cells break down, usually because of old age (red blood cells live only about 120 days). It is filtered out of the blood by the liver and altered into a more soluble form through a process called conjugation. That compound is then secreted into the bile and used as a digestive aid.

Your albumin and bilirubin levels are good indicators of your liver's efficiency and your overall good health.

What is cirrhosis?

Cirrhosis is scar tissue inside the liver that forms when liver cells are damaged or destroyed, as the liver attempts to repair itself. As cirrhosis progresses and scar tissue accumulates, blood vessels inside the liver are compressed and flow is obstructed, which can lead to deterioration of liver function and a number of complications. There is no single cause of cirrhosis. Among the major causes of cirrhosis are alcohol abuse; hepatitis B and C; autoimmune disease, which occurs when the body's immune system attacks the liver for reasons not clearly understood; and nonalcoholic steatohepatitis (NASH), a stage of nonalcoholic fatty liver disease, the most common liver disease in the United States.

Nearly twenty-eight thousand Americans die each year of cirrhosis, making it the fourth leading cause of death for people between the ages of forty-five and fifty-four, and the sixth leading cause of death for people between the ages of thirty-five and forty-four. However, if you are between the ages of twenty-five and thirty-four, you have not escaped the threat of cirrhosis—within that age group, it is the tenth leading cause of death.

One of the most insidious things about cirrhosis is the manner in which it progresses—and that is because it is an "either/or" disease. By that I mean that in its chronic state it can take years, even decades, to develop, existing in the body like a slow-burning ember, while in its later stages it can flame up like a raging fire and cause death within a relatively short period of time if not treated.

In its early stages, cirrhosis may produce no symptoms whatsoever. There are instances in which patients have unknowingly had the disease for twenty or thirty years. The early symptoms are usually mild and very subtle, and often they are attributed to other, less serious causes, such as indigestion.

The most important early symptoms are:

○ Diarrhea
○ Fatigue
○ Dull abdominal pain
○ Indigestion
○ Weight loss
○ Weakness
○ Vomiting
○ Loss of appetite
○ Musty breath

> *My doctor kept giving me medicine for one thing or another
> —high blood pressure, sinus infections, and so on—
> and each time I reported side effects he merely
> changed the medication. He never once mentioned
> that I could have cirrhosis, which is what I later discovered
> was the real reason for the side effects.
> I wish I had asked more questions.*
>
> —MARY P.

Almost every cirrhosis patient can look back and figure out when the disease began, but it is very difficult to do at the time these early symptoms occur because of the elusiveness of the symptoms. The oyster dinner that made you ill may be the result of assorted bacteria in the food—or it may be an early symptom of cirrhosis. That time you became ill after drinking too much could have been caused by the alcohol irritating your sensitive stomach lining—or it might have been an early symptom of cirrhosis. Those times you kept returning to your doctor because the medications he prescribed for you produced troublesome side effects may simply have been bad luck—or it may have been an early symptom of cirrhosis.

As the disease progresses, the symptoms become more alarming. Fluid may collect in your stomach or abdominal cavity (**ascites**) or in your legs (**edema**). Spiderlike blood vessels may appear on your chest and shoulders. Women may experience menstrual irregularities. Men may lose chest hair and grow breasts, and their testicles may shrink.

You may experience tremors, hallucinations, or memory loss. Since you do not know that you have a life-threatening disease, it is easy to rationalize the tremors as something that happens because you didn't get enough sleep. If you experience an auditory or visual hallucination, you may find it so frightening that you simply put it out of your mind and refuse to deal with it for fear you will be called crazy. And, of course, it is easy to rationalize memory loss as due to "getting older."

In the end-stage of the disease, the whites of the eyes and the skin become yellow because of the liver's inability to process bile from the gallbladder (by contrast, people with acute hepatitis turn yellow early in the disease); the urine turns dark yellow or brown; the skin is dry and itches for no apparent reason; and patients have problems sleeping, become forgetful, and have problems concentrating. As fewer toxins are filtered out by the liver and more enter the bloodstream, mental problems can become an issue. These are often evidenced by changes in behavior. Patients who were unconcerned about their appearance before the disease may become fastidious dressers—or the opposite may occur. Many of the mental problems associated with the disease may be so subtle as to be unnoticeable to people who have not known the patient for very long.

Of course, the goal in your treatment is to avoid the final stages of the disease. By taking an active role in your treatment, you increase your odds of doing just that. Cirrhosis is not a disease for which you can take a pill or undergo surgery. Successful treatment depends on dozens of small steps that you must take yourself.

IN A SENTENCE:

> *The first step to living with cirrhosis is understanding the disease and its symptoms.*

First Things First

When I got home from the doctor,
the first thing I did was clean out
the refrigerator. I threw everything out
except the fruit. Then I scrubbed
the refrigerator down with soap and water.

—TONYA B.

BEING TOLD that you have cirrhosis is not the final act in the drama of your life. It is the first act in the beginning of the rest of your life. You may feel that your life is out of control, but there is really no time to sit down and feel sorry for yourself.

You have work to do.

You have two choices: you can surrender to your disease—and experience an early death—or you can fight your disease by learning how to live with it. Being cured of cirrhosis is possible in some situations (the liver has a remarkable ability to regenerate tissue, although that does not mean that it can dispose of scar tissue), but, for the most part, cirrhosis is irreversible. Being a survivor means learning to cope with that patch of scar tissue on your liver for the rest of your life.

I am assuming that because you are reading this book, you do not want to surrender to your disease. Good for you! Much of your future is still in your hands. You are not powerless—you have the ability and the means to fight back. As Rolling Stone Mick Jagger sang early in his career, "You can make it if you try."

The first thing you will want to do when you get home from that devastating visit to your doctor's office is to take stock of your life and make a mental list of positive-action steps to gather strength. As a first step, I offer the following suggestions:

- Find a quiet place in your home. Sit down. If you have a dog or a cat that you care about, pick up your little friend and hold her in your lap.
- Pray for strength. If you are not religious, meditate on the words, "I am strong." As the saying goes, "It sure can't hurt."
- Cry if you feel the need to. You have earned the right.
- If you have a significant other, do not be hunkered down in a chair holding your cat when he or she arrives. Be on your feet at the door, looking like someone who is ready to embrace life—no matter how sorry you feel for yourself.

Make a checklist of action steps

Inner strength is more a by-product of *action* than determination. The reality is that you have a problem that you can't think your way out of. The solution requires action, not introspection. You may find it helpful to make a list of practical things that require immediate action on your part. Examples should include:

Vaccinations. It is extremely important that you schedule an appointment for a hepatitis vaccination. The type of vaccination you need will depend on the cause of your cirrhosis. If your disease resulted from hepatitis A, B, or C, then talk to your doctor about the advisability of being vaccinated for the types of hepatitis you do not have (there is no vaccination for hepatitis C). Vaccinations for hepatitis A and B can be administered separately or in a combined dosage. You also should receive a pneumococcal vaccine (Pneumovax) and a yearly flu shot.

Alcohol. From this day forward, there is no room for alcohol in your life—not if you want to survive this illness. Unless you are an alcoholic, you should be able to eliminate all alcoholic beverages from your diet immediately. If you are addicted to alcohol, no one will expect you to simply walk away from alcoholic beverages. In that case, it is important for you to find the help you need to terminate your dependency.

You should view alcohol as the poison that it is. It is your liver's responsibility to neutralize and then eliminate the poisons that enter your bloodstream. If your liver has been injured by cirrhosis and you continue to consume alcohol, you are asking your liver to perform a function that it cannot do with efficiency. Every drink you take is another week or so subtracted from your life.

Smoking. Whether you have already been thinking about it or not, now is the time for you to stop smoking. You may be one of those people who find cigarettes or cigars soothing. But please don't convince yourself that you need that cigarette or cigar as a crutch to help get you through the day. Replace it with something healthier that gives you pleasure. Cigarette smoke has been cited as a factor in causing liver cancer, and the fact that you have cirrhosis makes you more likely to develop liver cancer (more about that in Month 6). Quitting smoking is one of the best things you can do to dramatically decrease your risk.

Recreational drugs. This is a no-brainer. If you are using recreational drugs of any kind, stop. There is evidence that cocaine is toxic to the liver, especially when mixed with alcohol. There have been instances in which cocaine use among liver patients has led to premature death. Some research indicates that cocaine and ecstasy may actually cause hepatitis, which could be fatal to someone with cirrhosis. Marijuana has not been linked to hepatitis or liver cancer, but there is evidence that it decreases the effectiveness of some drug therapies and diminishes a patient's response to the medication. If you have cirrhosis, there is no "upside" to recreational drug use.

Sexual activity. If you are in a stable sexual relationship, you should have your partner tested for hepatitis B. About 50 percent of partners tested show evidence of past exposure, so they do not need to be vaccinated or change their sexual practices. For nonexposed partners, vaccination is critical. For patients with multiple partners, safe sex practices are essential. For people with hepatitis C who are in stable relationships, the risk of sexual transmission is low, unless either partner has genital herpes, genital warts, or bleeding with intercourse. .

"The incidence of sexual transmission of hepatitis C is very low, and most such cases likely stem from a mingling of blood during sexual contact," says Dr. Melissa Palmer, author of *Hepatitis and Liver Disease*, who adds, "It appears that it is easier to transmit hepatitis C from men to women than vice versa."

Since the hepatitis virus is carried in blood, cirrhosis patients should not engage in vaginal or oral intercourse while the woman is having her period; nor is it advisable for cirrhosis patients to engage in anal intercourse because of the possibility of bleeding.

Stress. One of your worst enemies for the duration of your disease will be stress, for the simple reason that stress prevents your immune system from doing its job. It is important for you to take stock of your life and identify the major sources of stress that you experience on a regular basis. This is one area where you must be vigilant. If you have personal and business relationships that cause you stress, you should reexamine those relationships and distance yourself from the ones that do not offer a compensating upside. Tolerating a stressful relationship is a ticket to an early grave.

If you are having marital problems, I am not suggesting that you rush out and get a divorce. What I am suggesting is that you take a close look at your relationship. If you have been experiencing serious problems in your relationship, it is likely that your diagnosis will only exacerbate those problems. Now is the time for you to seek professional help in resolving the issues associated with your relationship.

If *things*, not people, are what cause you stress, you must engage in some creative problem solving. For example, if leaky plumbing is causing you stress, then do whatever it takes to solve that problem— or resolve to "let go" of allowing it to bother you. If you are constantly thinking, *I just hate that the sink keeps dripping, but can't possibly deal with a plumber, not when I'm fighting for my life*, then you are missing the point. Fighting for your life is directly related to how well you handle the many small stresses in your life. So, if plumbing is what causes you stress, pick up the phone book and make that call! Or, decide that you can live with a leaky faucet. Be a doer, not a complainer, and watch as your entire outlook gets more positive.

Exercise. One of the characteristics of liver disease is a lack of energy. A good way to counteract that is to exercise. That may sound paradoxical, but it works because it improves cardiovascular function and that leads to more energy. Exercise also reduces body fat, an important consideration because excess body fat puts a strain on the liver and makes it more difficult for it to do its job. If you establish a regular exercise routine, you will find that the benefits will be worth it.

IN A SENTENCE:

Healthier lifestyle choices will empower you to take charge of your treatment.

learning

How Your Liver Works

Not long after I was diagnosed with cirrhosis
I went to a restaurant with my husband.
I noticed that the gentleman sitting at the next table
was eating liver and I just snapped.
"How can you do that?" I demanded.
The idea of him eating an organ that valuable
just made me crazy.

—MELINDA H.

WE HAVE already discussed where the liver is located. We have gone over its purpose and looked at how important this organ is to your survival. Now let's examine in more detail how it works.

In order to cleanse your body of toxic substances, the liver takes a factorylike approach to its work. It gathers compounds such as toxins, nutrients, and drugs from your blood and re-directs each to its proper place like one of those automated mail-sorting machines used by the post office. The compounds are moved along through specialized capillaries called sinusoids. Since the sinusoids are permeable, they enable the drugs, nutri-ents, and toxins picked up by the blood to have access to the liver's major cells, the **hepatocytes**, which metabolize the com-pounds so that they can be processed by the body's other organs.

That process allows toxins to be cleansed from the blood and secreted into small bile ducts that combine to form the common bile duct that channels into the small intestine. Bile is composed of many compounds, including salts, cholesterol, fatty acids, and a pigment called bilirubin.

Bilirubin

Bilirubin is the equivalent of the canary-in-a-cage that miners once carried with them into a mine shaft, the idea being that the bird would die if the air was unfit for humans. Bilirubin is the body's early warning sign. A greenish yellow substance, it is made from chemically converted hemoglobin, the protein that carries oxygen in the blood.

Your bilirubin level is a good indicator of your liver's efficiency. If your liver is damaged, for whatever reason, bilirubin will accumulate in your blood and make your skin and the whites of your eyes look yellow (jaundiced). If, for some reason, your liver is not secreting bilirubin into the bile, your urine will appear dark yellow or brown.

Normally your urine will be almost clear, with a very light yellow or straw color. There are several relatively benign reasons why your urine may be dark or bright yellow (you may not be drinking enough water, for example), but it can also indicate serious liver problems, such as the inflammation that causes cirrhosis.

If you have cirrhosis, your urine color will let you know if your liver is undergoing important changes. If it goes from light to dark and stays that way for several days, you should notify your doctor, since it could indicate a worsening of your condition and your doctor will probably want to order tests to evaluate the bilirubin levels in your blood. If your urine goes from dark to light, that might be an indication that the source of your cirrhosis is no longer advancing.

Albumin

Albumin, which is secreted by the liver, is the most plentiful protein in your blood. There are many reasons why a person's albumin levels may be low—kidney disease, for example, or improper nutrition, or poor health in general—but one of the most disturbing reasons is liver damage. People with damaged livers often have low levels of albumin in their blood.

Your doctor will be concerned about low albumin levels in your blood because the absence of the protein can aggravate fluid buildups known as ascites and edema.

Blood clotting

If it were not for your liver manufacturing the clotting agents that the body uses to stop bleeding, you would bleed to death from minor cuts. Vitamin K is an important factor in blood clotting, and if the liver is damaged so that it cannot store sufficient amounts of the vitamin, uncontrolled bleeding can become a serious issue.

Blood clotting is complicated. Prothrombin time measures one aspect of the clotting cascade, but it does not measure the platelets' ability to clot. Platelet number and function also contribute to the clotting mechanism. A prolonged prothrombin time is not related to platelets. When blood is shunted to the spleen, you may get low platelets, but that is unrelated to prothrombin time.

Normally clots form in nine to eleven seconds. A clotting time longer than that may be an indication of the severity of your cirrhosis and it may simply mean that your vitamin K levels are unusually low. Faced with an extended clotting time, your doctor may give you a vitamin K injection as a way to test your liver function. If your clotting time improves dramatically after you receive the vitamin K, it is an indication that your liver is still working. If your clotting time does not improve after the injection, it may indicate that your liver is stressed and headed toward total failure.

Ammonia

When amino acid breaks down in the body, it produces a toxic substance called ammonia. It is the liver's job to remove ammonia from the bloodstream. If the liver is unable to remove the ammonia, due to cirrhosis or some other liver problem, the toxin circulates unfiltered through the bloodstream.

Some doctors feel that ammonia levels in the blood correlate with a form of brain damage called **encephalopathy**, but others point out that research has failed to connect specific ammonia levels with encephalopathy. Actually, ammonia is one of a number of toxins that can contribute to the development of encephalopathy. Ammonia is the only one that can routinely be measured, which is why people think there is a direct relationship between ammonia and encephalopathy. One thing most doctors are able to agree on is that toxic buildups in the blood can cause confusion, sleepiness, and even coma in some people.

Cholesterol

Your liver is the only organ in your body that removes cholesterol from your bloodstream. It does that by filtering it out of your blood and then converting it into bile acids that are essential for the digestion of fats.

When your liver does not do its job properly, the fatty buildup creates gallstones and releases the fatty cells back into the bloodstream, where they clog the arteries. As with all other functions, the liver's ability to filter cholesterol is adversely affected by cirrhosis, which is one reason why cirrhosis patients are prone to gallstones.

The relationship between cirrhosis and high cholesterol is often overlooked by doctors not accustomed to treating liver disease. In fairness, that is because few cases of high cholesterol are an indicator of liver damage, and many doctors find comfort in playing the odds when they make a diagnosis. However, it would save lives if doctors who encountered high cholesterol in their patients also looked for other indicators of cirrhosis—hemorrhoids, mild indigestion, high blood pressure, an intolerance to drugs, and slow clotting—before writing a prescription to treat the symptom of high cholesterol.

Estrogen

Estrogen is one of two major classes of female hormones—progestins being the second class—that are metabolized by the liver. As you are probably aware, small levels of estrogen are also present in males. When the liver fails to process estrogen properly, it presents different problems for males and females.

In males, faulty estrogen processing in the liver can cause **gynecomastia**, an enlargement of the breast. It can occur in one breast or in both breasts. Not all male breast enlargement is related to cirrhosis—sometimes the process begins at puberty and relates to the balance of estrogen and testosterone; other times it is related to undiscovered tumors or drug reactions, and can occur at any age—but it is a fairly reliable indicator of cirrhosis in males, especially when other symptoms are evident. In rare cases, it can lead to male breast cancer.

In females, faulty estrogen processing in the liver can result in high blood pressure, premenstrual syndrome (PMS), and breast and vaginal cancer. It is not known whether estrogen is involved or not, but a common complaint of women with cirrhosis is that their breasts are shrinking.

IN A SENTENCE:

> *An efficient liver works in many ways to process nutrients, toxins, and chemicals, keeping you healthy.*

living

Finding the Right Doctors

ONCE A primary care physician has given you an initial diagnosis of cirrhosis, he or she may refer you to a gastro-enterologist for further testing and treatment. While your new doctor is sizing up your disease in an effort to determine its cause and severity, you will be sizing up your doctor to decide if he or she is the right person to direct your treatment. At some point, your gastroenterologist will probably refer you to a physician who specializes in liver diseases (a hepatologist).

All doctors are not created equal, which is why finding the right one is not as easy as it might seem. You may get lucky and find an extremely qualified, available, attentive doctor right away. Or it may take some time to find one with whom you are comfortable and who matches your needs and budget. As you read in the introduction, I had an unpleasant experience with a doctor early in my illness and I had to be aggressive in my efforts to find a replacement. But eventually, I found two great doctors—and I couldn't be happier with them.

Unless you were diagnosed with a chronic illness before learning that you have cirrhosis, the odds are that you have gone through most of your life without giving much thought to your physicians. If you are like most people, you have changed jobs and moved to different cities several times. With each move you have had to find a new primary care doctor when you became ill—and that was probably for minor illnesses such as the flu or indigestion or allergies, or for the treatment of minor cuts.

You have probably liked some doctors better than others, tolerating the ones you didn't like because they were convenient to your home or office. When I was very young, I once went to a doctor when I had a sore throat. He was a crusty old soul, but he came highly recommended. I asked him if he thought my sore throat might be due to cancer. His curt response was, "Well, it's either cancer and you'll die, or it's an infection that will go away in a week or so." My sore throat wasn't cancer, and it went away within a week.

I should have moved on to another physician after he took such a cavalier attitude to my question, but I didn't because I liked him as a person, I was young and he had years of experience—and he was *right*, after all. A year or so after that, he delivered my son, missing my wife's toxemia in the weeks leading up to the delivery, an oversight that nearly cost her her life when her blood pressure soared to stroke levels.

Later, that same doctor, when told that our son would not stop crying, advised us to not pick him up. "Just let him cry," he said. "He'll get tired of it eventually." Again, he missed the mark. As it turned out, my son had a hernia that was causing him great pain. After that event, we found a new family physician and a pediatrician for our son.

My advice to you is to enter a relationship with a new doctor with an open-minded attitude; do trust that they have your best interests at heart. However, do not hesitate to move on if the doctor is not responsive to your questions or if he or she misdiagnoses your illness. That is especially true if you have been diagnosed with a chronic disease such as cirrhosis. You need a medical team who will stick with you for the rest of your life (or his or her life), however long that might be.

At this point in your treatment, you may not know enough about cirrhosis—or your particular condition—to ask your doctor detailed questions about your disease. What you can do is evaluate the doctor's response to you as a person. Was enough time spent explaining the basics of the disease and the treatment plan? Was there eye contact with you during your examination? Were you encouraged to ask questions? Most important, when you left the doctor's office, did you feel that you were in good hands?

What kinds of doctors treat liver disease?

Your introduction to cirrhosis was probably not from a specialist in liver disease. Most likely, you went to a family physician with complaints of dark urine, jaundice, or mild stomach distress—or you may have gone to your primary care physician for your annual physical, only to be told that your routine blood tests revealed a potential problem.

Family physicians, general practitioners, and primary care physicians generally do not attempt to diagnosis cirrhosis. If they strongly suspect that a patient has cirrhosis, they refer the patient to a gastroenterologist or to a hepatologist (if one is available; they are scarce in rural areas) so that a diagnosis can be made by a doctor who is familiar with the disease. Some people think that a doctor is a doctor and it doesn't matter whether you see a specialist or not. Others find the different medical labels confusing. Hopefully this section will help you clarify your stance.

> **General practitioner.** This is a medical doctor who has completed four years of medical school training. After leaving medical school, general practitioners are required to complete a minimum of one year of training in a hospital. Before practicing medicine, they must pass a state licensing examination.
>
> **Primary care physician.** The most common types of PCPs are internists, family physicians, pediatricians, and obstetrician/gynecologists. They act as the primary gatekeepers of the medical profession by determining when patients should be referred to specialists.
>
> **The family physician.** A medical doctor is someone who has graduated from medical school and then completed a minimum of one year of additional training in a hospital as an intern. A family physician is a medical doctor who has undergone an additional two years of training beyond an internship. Upon completion of their training, family physicians are required to be certified by a family practice board (thus the term *board certified*). If they pass the examination, they can call themselves family practitioners. Their focus is general in nature and includes training in gynecology, obstetrics, psychiatry, and surgery. However, they do not undergo any specialized training in liver disease.

The internist. This is a medical doctor who has received two years of training beyond an internship in subspecialty areas of internal medicine such as infectious diseases, hepatology, or gastroenterology. Since internists have the option of continuing their training in a specific area, some choose to focus on liver diseases. The only way to know your internist's specialty is to ask.

The gastroenterologist. This is an internist who has received special training in the treatment of digestive disorders involving the esophagus, small and large intestines, stomach, pancreas, gallbladder, and liver. To be certified as a gastroenterologist, the doctor must first be certified in internal medicine and then undergo an additional two or three years of study beyond his or her residency in internal medicine. Some gastroenterologists receive little training in liver diseases, while others focus on that area. The only way to know if your gastroenterologist has training in liver diseases is to ask.

The hepatologist. This is the person most qualified to treat people with liver disease. Unlike many other medical specialties, hepatology does not have a separate board certification process. A doctor becomes a hepatologist by receiving special training under a fellowship that usually lasts up to two years. Most, but not all, hepatologists are gastroenterologists. Any internist who receives specialized training in liver disease is considered a hepatologist. If you have cirrhosis, you will want a hepatologist involved in your treatment, whether it is as the primary caregiver or as a consultant. In my case, I chose a gastroenterologist who lives in my hometown and a hepatologist in another city who is involved with a university hospital's liver transplant center.

Infectious disease specialist. This is an internist who has completed a specialty fellowship in infectious diseases. If the cause of your cirrhosis is hepatitis, you may have an infectious disease specialist involved in your treatment. However, if he or she has no special training in diseases of the liver, you probably will not want him or her to be your primary care physician.

Academic physicians vs. private practitioners

Once you have decided on a specialist, you must decide whether you want your doctor to be a private practitioner or affiliated with a university. A private practitioner is a doctor who focuses his efforts on patient care in a private setting, whether as part of a group practice in which there are several partners in the same field or in an individual practice in which other doctors are not involved.

An academic physician is one who has a faculty position at a university hospital. These doctors teach medical students and oversee interns, residents, and fellows while they complete requirements for their specialty, but they also treat patients on an individual basis. Such doctors come with positive and negative aspects. Since they also spend a great deal of time attending conferences and lectures, academic practitioners usually require their patients to make appointments weeks or months in advance. That is a negative consideration for patients who require a lot of personal attention.

On the positive side, academic practitioners are the first to hear about new treatments and they are often involved in clinical trials for new medications, a consideration that may prove to be important to you if traditional treatments fail to slow the progress of your cirrhosis.

In the end, whether you choose a private practitioner or an academic physician will probably depend on your location and the availability of specialists in your city. It will also depend on your personality (do you require a lot of personal attention, or can you go weeks or months without contact with your doctor and not be stressed?) and on your expectations for long-term treatment.

Second opinions

You shouldn't be hesitant to seek out a second opinion if you have been diagnosed with cirrhosis, but you should make certain that the doctor you are asking for a second opinion has the same or better qualifications than the one who made your original diagnosis. Also, you should be honest with yourself. Is it a second opinion that you want? Or is it a denial that you have cirrhosis? If it is the latter, rest assured that if you see enough doctors you eventually will find one who gives you a different diagnosis.

Of course, if you have two or three specialists telling you that you have cirrhosis—and one doctor who says you don't—common sense dictates that you should accept the possibility that the lone dissenter may be mistaken.

Above all else, use good judgment. Cirrhosis is not a disease that can be ignored for very long. If you delay treatment, you may find that you have waited too long.

IN A SENTENCE:

> *Devote as much time and effort to selecting doctors as you need to feel comfortable.*

learning

Understanding the Medical Tests You Will Be Given

IN THE days and weeks after your initial cirrhosis diagnosis, your physician will run further tests to evaluate how well your liver is functioning. In the beginning, your journey into the world of liver disease may seem intimidating and overwhelming. If you have been relatively healthy for most of your life, you will hear the names of tests and procedures that will be new to you.

You may even experience performance anxiety. Of course, you want to cooperate in every way possible, but what if you do something "wrong" that causes you to "fail" the test? What if you hold your arm wrong? What if you don't take a deep enough breath? How can you do well on a test if you don't understand the test?

Doctors seldom explain the tests they are ordering for you unless you ask, so if you have questions, don't be afraid to speak up. Don't let your imagination run wild as you try to figure out what kind of experience you are headed for based on the name of the test!

The good news is that none of the tests you will be asked to take depend on your participation to any great degree. Undergoing the tests and procedures is a little like riding up an escalator. You just get comfortable and wait for the procedure to move you from point A to point B. The technicians and nurses involved will take care of the rest. They won't ask you to do anything difficult. You'll hear things like, "Hold your breath, please," or "Turn on your side, please." In all likelihood, a needle prick will be the only slightly painful experience you receive, but even this is over very quickly.

Your doctors should make you aware of any tests that have potential side effects because of radiation involved. Of course, the risks are usually minimal, and if your doctor thinks you may have cirrhosis or some other liver disease, he or she is not going to hesitate to order the tests for you. Remember, the risks to you are much greater if you don't have the tests. It can be frustrating to go through this when you're not used to being a patient, but try to get used to the fact that you are now living in a new world!

Blood tests

The first tests your doctor orders are likely to be liver function tests (LFTs). The name is misleading, in a way, because it doesn't provide information on how the liver is functioning as a whole, only on how parts of the liver are functioning. As a result, each test result is like a jigsaw puzzle piece, one small part of the whole picture.

> **Liver enzymes.** Four different liver enzymes are measured on most liver function tests—**aspartate aminotransferase** (**AST** or **SGOT**), **alanine aminotransferase** (**ALT** or **SGPT**), **alkaline phosphatase** (**AP**), and **gamma-glutamyl transferase** (**GGTP**). Elevated levels of these enzymes are associated with inflammation or injury to liver cells, although they can be due to other causes, such as muscle disorders.
>
> If AST levels are higher than ALT levels, that may tell the doctor that cirrhosis is present. If ALT levels are higher than AST levels, that might be indicative of liver disease other than cirrhosis.
>
> Enzyme tests are an important diagnostic tool, but they are not definitive in determining whether you have liver disease. Men normally have higher scores than women. African-American men usually have higher

scores than Caucasian men. Levels are often higher in the morning and afternoon than they are in the evening. One alcoholic drink consumed a couple of hours before the test can skew the results.

To complicate matters, if the liver was damaged several years before the blood test was given, the enzyme levels may test in the normal range. High levels of the tested enzymes may indicate liver disease, but low or normal levels do not necessarily indicate the absence of liver disease.

Complete blood count. This test allows the doctor to determine if your red blood cells and white blood cells are within normal ranges. Liver disease patients often have a normal or a low red blood count (a condition called anemia). Their white blood count can be low, high, or normal. This test is not used to pinpoint the cause of your problem, but rather to gauge your overall health.

Bilirubin. As discussed earlier, this is the yellow-colored pigment that most people associate with liver disease since it may turn the patient's skin and eyes yellow. Elevated bilirubin levels are often associated with cirrhosis or other liver diseases, but this test is not definitive for cirrhosis since there can be other reasons for the elevation. Causes other than cirrhosis include: viral hepatitis, tumors on the liver or gallbladder, gallstones in the bile duct, and drug-induced liver disease. If you are being treated for cirrhosis, your doctor will be interested in your bilirubin level because if it is going up, that may indicate that you are not responding to treatment as well as expected. If it is going down, it may indicate that the inflammation in your liver is cooling somewhat.

Prothrombin time. This is the blood test that measures your clotting time. Normally it takes the body nine to eleven seconds to form a clot, but if the liver has undergone significant damage, that clotting time will be extended beyond eleven seconds. A normal prothrombin time is an indication that your cirrhosis has not affected this important function. A prothrombin time of longer than eleven seconds may indicate that your cirrhosis is progressing toward complications that will require your doctor's attention.

Albumin. A low albumin level is consistent with overall poor health and is not specific to liver disease. However, cirrhosis is usually accompanied by a low albumin level and your doctor will use your albumin level as yet another piece of the puzzle he or she is putting together for your diagnosis.

Alpha-fetoprotein (AFP). This test is used to screen for a specific liver tumor called **primary hepatocellular carcinoma**. Having a high AFP level does not mean you have a tumor, since other factors can cause it to rise, but a low AFP level provides your doctor with more confidence that a tumor does not exist.

Serum ceruloplasmin. This test will be ordered by your doctor if he or she suspects that you might have **Wilson's disease**, a condition associated with excessive amounts of copper in the body.

Hepatitis viral serological markers. These are tests that are used to look for the hepatitis viruses. There is a separate test for each type of hepatitis—A, B, and C.

Sonograms (ultrasound)

Sonograms are the most common imaging tests used to evaluate the liver. This is the test that is so familiar to pregnant women, the one that provides the mother with her first look at the baby inside her womb. It is a popular screening device because it is a relatively quick and inexpensive way to evaluate certain aspects of the liver. It is also popular because it uses sound waves instead of radiation and therefore poses no side-effect risk to the patient.

What the sonogram can and cannot do:

○ It can detect gallstones.
○ It can detect masses on the liver, but it cannot determine whether they are benign or cancerous.
○ It can estimate the size of a mass on the liver.
○ It can detect the buildup of fluids (ascites) around the liver.
○ It cannot detect cirrhosis per se, but it can identify features associated with cirrhosis (fluid retention in the abdominal cavity, for example).

A sonogram is a painless procedure. You will be asked to take off your shirt and lie down on an examining table. The technician will apply a sticky gel over your abdomen and then he or she will move a device called a transducer over your skin while watching the images on a video screen. When the technician sees something of interest, he or she will manipulate a keyboard and save those images so that they can later be printed out on paper and evaluated by a radiologist. Often you will be asked to move about and lie on each side so that the technician can get a better view of your liver.

The liver-spleen scan

This is a nuclear test that is used to detect cirrhosis in its later stages. It involves injecting a radioactive compound into the patient's bloodstream and then photographing the radiation with a special camera. If the patient has moderate or advanced cirrhosis, the radioactive compound will be shunted to the spleen or taken in by the bone marrow, both of which activities can be picked up by the camera. This test will not detect cirrhosis in its early stages.

CT (or CAT) scan

The CT, or CAT (computed axial tomography), scan is the heavy hitter of all X-ray devices. Instead of sending a single X-ray through your body, it uses a computer to send numerous X-rays through your body simultaneously at different angles. The computer takes those images and creates a three-dimensional picture that is displayed on a monitor.

During this process, the patient is asked to lie on a table that is moved into a cylinder that allows the X-ray machine to move around the patient. Prior to beginning the process, the patient will be given an injection containing a dye. In rare cases, the dye has been known to cause allergic reactions and to damage already weakened kidneys.

Unlike the sonogram, the CT scan exposes the patient to significant amounts of radiation and for that reason should not be used on patients who do not have symptoms of serious disease. For patients with symptoms of serious disease, however, the CT scan can be a lifesaver, especially in those situations when it detects malignant tumors that otherwise have not revealed themselves.

Pluses and minuses of the CT scan:

○ It can display cross-sections of the liver.
○ It can detect features associated with more advanced cirrhosis (nodular liver, ascites, varices, etc.), but it cannot detect the disease per se.

- ○ It can detect liver tumors.
- ○ It has been known to produce inaccurate "normal" findings.
- ○ It has been known to produce false positives, which have led to unnecessary additional testing.

The important thing to remember about the CT scan is that it is not going to give you a definitive report on the health of your liver. Keep that in mind when you receive the results of your CT scan—don't despair if they are negative and don't jump for joy if they are positive. In my case, a CT scan detected no abnormalities in my liver. It totally missed my cirrhosis. If my doctor had formed a conclusion based on the CT scan, he would have sent me home with a diagnosis of good health. He was too good a doctor to do that, and he pressed on and asked me to undergo the most definitive test available for liver disease—the biopsy. A biopsy, in which cell and tissue samples are removed from the liver for analysis, is the final step in the diagnostic process and the only test that can definitively detect cirrhosis. As this is a more serious procedure, I discuss this test in detail in Week 2.

Endoscopic evaluation

In this test, a lighted instrument, called an endoscope, is lowered down your throat and into your stomach, or possibly as far as the upper part of your small intestine, to allow visual inspection of your esophagus, stomach, and bile and pancreatic ducts. It is used to identify conditions that will be of interest in treating your cirrhosis. A procedure called spontaneous peritonitis sclerotherapy may be used; it involves the injection of a chemical solution into varicose veins in your esophagus made visible by the endoscope. An additional step may involve the injection of dye into the bile and pancreatic ducts so that X-rays can be taken to identify problem areas.

IN A SENTENCE:

> *After the initial diagnosis, further medical tests are essential to confirm a diagnosis and determine the condition of your liver.*

How Did I Get This Disease?

ONE DAY you are doing great. The next day you are told that you have a life-threatening disease. This is, understandably, a very difficult notion to grapple with, and many people look at their illness as a mystery to be solved. In the case of cirrhosis, working with your physician to determine what has caused your condition can be essential to your future treatment. To that end, it's vital to be honest when answering your physician's questions about your health history.

Your physician probably will not ask you about your sexual orientation, in keeping with the political correctness of the times, but if you are gay it may be in your best interest to disclose that fact since it could be helpful in pinpointing the cause of your cirrhosis (homosexuals are a high-risk group). And no matter what your sexual orientation, you should alert your physician if you have had unprotected sex. Your physician will want to know if you have a drinking problem or abuse drugs. Again, it is essential that you answer honestly. Your life may depend on it.

When Suze G. was told she had cirrhosis, she was stunned but not entirely surprised. She had been a closet alcoholic for more than twenty years, hiding her drinking problem from loved ones and friends, who never saw her take more than one drink at a time. In truth, she consumed a fifth of vodka each day.

Suze was asked point-blank by her doctor how much alcohol she consumed.

"Maybe I'll average a couple of drinks a week," she lied, embarrassed.

Faced with a convincing patient, the physician redirected her efforts into exploring other possible causes of Suze's cirrhosis, a process that took weeks of costly testing and examinations. By the time Suze finally admitted that she had a drinking problem, she had begun experiencing serious complications from cirrhosis.

Learn from Suze's mistake: be honest with your doctor!

Among the many causes of cirrhosis are:

○ **Hepatitis B.** You may have contracted the disease through a blood transfusion, or from bodily fluids such as urine, tears, semen, or vaginal or breast secretions—or from a minor cut, or IV drug use, or a toothbrush or even from a kiss. Tattoos, ear or body piercing, and dental work are other means of transmission. Hepatitis B is a frequent cause of cirrhosis.

○ **Hepatitis C.** You may have been exposed to the disease through contaminated blood, IV drug use, recreational drug use, tattoos and body piercings, or sexual contact with an infected person. Hepatitis C is one of the most common causes of cirrhosis.

○ **Alcohol consumption.** In the United States, chronic alcohol consumption is the number-one cause of cirrhosis. If you are a heavy drinker, alcohol would have to be the primary suspect.

○ **Prescription medications.** Your cirrhosis may have been caused by medications prescribed for a totally unrelated condition. "The actual number of drugs that cause cirrhosis is very small," says Dr. Fredric Regenstein. "But in the absence of other known causes of cirrhosis, drugs always need to be considered." Many drugs can cause liver damage or even hepatitis, but the most common categories are antibiotics, blood pressure medications, cholesterol medications, and analgesics such as acetaminophen (Tylenol) and ibuprofen (Motrin). Neither Tylenol nor Motrin have been demonstrated to cause cirrhosis, but Tylenol, when ingested in excessive amounts, can cause hepatitis and fulminant hepatic failure, conditions you want to avoid if you already have cirrhosis.

○ **Vitamins.** If you took large doses of vitamin A or other vitamins at some point in your life, it may have triggered your cirrhosis.

○ **Your genetics.** As explained earlier, autoimmune hepatitis is not a form of viral hepatitis, but rather a condition that is caused when your body attacks your liver because it considers it to be an invading organism. The end result is cirrhosis. Many doctors consider a genetic predisposition to the disease to be a primary factor. Wilson's disease, another genetic disorder, is associated with an overload of copper in the body, a condition that results in cirrhosis.

○ **Your diet.** Antibiotics and hormones given to cattle and poultry can cause liver damage in humans, but they are an unproven cause of cirrhosis. A more important dietary cause of cirrhosis is NASH, which is very much related to diet (carbs, fats, too many calories), the epidemic of obesity and diabetes, and a sedentary lifestyle.

As you can see from the above, some of the causes of cirrhosis are totally within your control, while others are not. In the days to come, I'll be going over the most common causes of cirrhosis in more depth. If your disease was caused by your behavior, remember that there is nothing you can do about it now and it will not be to your benefit to dwell on the "what ifs" of your life. On the other hand, there *is* plenty you can do from this point on to increase your chances of recovery—and *that* should be the focus of your thoughts—not the past.

IN A SENTENCE:

Establishing the cause of your cirrhosis is important because it determines your treatment.

learning

Breaking the News to Loved Ones

What I remember most about the day
I was told I had cirrhosis was not
my own reaction, but my husband's
stunned look of disbelief. For weeks afterward,
I saw that face every night in my dreams.

—HARRIET M.

IN MANY ways, telling others that you have cirrhosis is more difficult than hearing the news yourself from your doctor. That's because listening to bad news is a passive event, while giving bad news to others requires your active participation. Often the realization that you have a life-threatening disease will not be fully felt until you say the words yourself.

The "telling" process is doubly difficult if you have a disease that is associated, at least in the public mind, with alcohol or substance abuse, or with sexual misbehavior of various kinds. In that sense, cirrhosis often carries the same stigma as HIV and hepatitis.

Deciding when and if to disclose your condition to others is completely up to you, and you may wish to wait until the details of your diagnosis and treatment plan are more clear. That said, you'll probably want to tell your closest loved ones right away. Whether that is a significant other, your parents, your children, or your close friends, is entirely up to you. A great deal will depend on your relationship with them. If you feel a little shaky, you will want to divide your loved-ones list into categories of who is likely to be supportive and who is not. At the top of your list should be those individuals who will be able to be sympathetic and supportive without falling apart.

Telling significant others

Your relationship with your significant other will determine how you tell them about your diagnosis. If possible, you should avoid doing it over the telephone, though that is not always possible, since your partner will know that you went to see a doctor and will be anxious to hear from you.

When you tell your partner or spouse, try to be as positive as you can, even though you may be feeling otherwise. A person's reaction to news tends to reflect the way they hear it. What you don't want to do is to tell your partner, "The doctor said I have cirrhosis"—and then break into tears without any further explanation. Instead, gather the breath for a long sentence and say, "The doctor said I have cirrhosis, but he was very encouraging about my prognosis" (as long as this is indeed the case).

Your partner will probably respond with something like, "What does that mean?"

The important thing for you to keep in mind—and to address in the initial moments of telling—is that your partner will have questions that he or she may be hesitant to ask. It is up to you to answer them before they are asked.

These are the questions that your partner will want to ask, and that you should be prepared to answer:

- "Are you going to die [right away]?"
- "Is this something that I can catch from you?"
- "How did you get it?"

The answer to the first question is almost always no, unless your doctor told you that you are in the midst of acute liver failure. Even then, there is time for you to be placed on a liver transplant waiting list, although there is no guarantee that you will receive a liver in time. As far as the other two questions are concerned, the answer depends on the cause of your cirrhosis. While cirrhosis itself is not contagious and cannot be transmitted to others, some of the causes of cirrhosis can be transmitted to others.

One of the things you will have to deal with is the fact that cirrhosis gets some of the worst PR of any disease I can think of, other than perhaps AIDS. The average person associates cirrhosis with alcoholics and IV drug users—and it is true that alcoholic liver disease and hepatitis C are the two most common causes of cirrhosis in the United States—but it is statistically difficult to link hepatitis C cases with IV drug use since the disease has many other causes. However, these are issues that you will have to deal with, especially if either scenario is applicable to your case.

If your cirrhosis was caused by hepatitis B or C, the result of drug abuse or an illicit affair, your partner is at risk of contracting the disease, and they should be told immediately so that they can be tested and then receive the proper vaccinations, if they do not have an active case of the disease.

If you are an alcoholic, whether you have admitted it to yourself yet or not, it is an issue that will have to be addressed in terms of your cirrhosis. Perhaps this has been a troublesome issue between you and your partner for a long time. If so, your partner may insist that you face up to your problem—or lose his or her support.

If you are an IV drug user, or used drugs in your distant past—and have kept that a secret from your partner—you will have to deal not only with the drug use, but with the deception—two separate issues that may affect your relationship in negative ways.

Because of the perception people have of cirrhosis, you may find yourself on the defensive when explaining your diagnosis. Your partner will be upset that you are ill, but he or she may also be angry that you have a disease that is identified with alcohol and drug use, which is likely to make you angry in return, because you feel that you already have enough to deal with without your partner initiating a blame game.

Of course, if your cirrhosis was not caused by alcohol or drug use, or an illicit affair, the phrase you will most often find yourself saying is, "I have cirrhosis, but it is not the type caused by alcohol or drug use—and I certainly haven't had an affair."

You have a right to expect unqualified support from your spouse, since that is the person you will lean on most for support, but you must understand that receiving that support is a two-way exchange that requires honesty from you about the cause of your cirrhosis. Also, you must face the fact that your partner may require time to fully digest the bad news and to come to terms with his or her role in your recovery.

Telling parents

It is important for you to be gentle with your parents. You want their sympathy, love, and support, but you don't want it to come at the expense of their own health, so you should focus on the encouraging aspects of your diagnosis—and there will be many.

Their reaction to your diagnosis should not be a surprise to you. This is probably not the first crisis you have shared with them, so don't expect your parents to behave in a new and creative way. If they have responded to past crises, even if it involved only broken hearts or financial setbacks, in a supportive, loving manner, chances are this one will be no different. If they tend to react with denial, anger, or benign neglect, you should be prepared for them to respond that way to the news of your disease.

If your cirrhosis is the result of alcohol or drug abuse, then you should be prepared for their anger. They may fear the worst—and the slightest possibility of that could dredge up deep feelings that may be more than they can handle at first. They may blame you for your illness—something you will not be in a frame of mind to hear. If your cirrhosis was caused by hepatitis, then you will have to talk to your parents about how they should protect themselves from the disease.

Once the first rush of emotions has come and gone, you will want to explain to your parents that, whatever the cause of your disease, it is not necessarily a death sentence. Explain to them that although your life will undergo some immediate changes, especially involving your diet, cirrhosis is a chronic disease that may not be life threatening for many years. You might want to say something like, "Mom and Dad, I know you're concerned, and your support means so much to me right now. I want you to know that my condition, though not curable, is treatable, and not necessarily life threatening. I'm going to be doing everything I can to improve my health. Try not to worry too much—for now, why don't we just relax and enjoy each other's company?"

Telling your children

When you tell your children should depend on their age. In my opinion, protecting young children is more important than telling them. No one knows your children better than you do, and you know their limits when it comes to bad news.

There is a difference between lying to your children and simply telling them less than you know. A general rule is that the older the child, the more you can tell them. For example, I can see no benefits to telling a five-year-old that you have cirrhosis. As they will have no prior knowledge of the disease, they will not be able to comprehend the seriousness of your situation. Second, unlike you, five-year-olds don't have different levels of fear. They are either afraid or they are not. You have tempered your fear of the disease with encouraging information that gives you hope for the future. Your child will have the fear, but not the hope, since they have not yet learned the perimeters of hope.

If your cirrhosis is the result of hepatitis C, you will need to take steps to protect your children from an infectious disease. That will entail gathering up any articles in your home that could have microscopic traces of your blood—razors, scissors, nail clippers, toothbrushes, etc., and keeping them out of your child's reach. Of course, you will want to explain to your children why such articles are dangerous to them. Just be very specific and tailor your comments to your child's age and maturity level.

Telling others

There is no law that requires you to notify your employer that you have cirrhosis, so whether you disclose that fact will depend on the nature of your working relationship. The Americans with Disabilities Act prohibits employers with fifteen or more employees from discriminating against individuals with disabilities, but it is unlikely that you will qualify as a disabled individual until you experience serious complications from your cirrhosis—and that could be years in the future, if at all.

If you work for a company with fewer than fifteen employees, or if your disease has not progressed to serious complications, it may be in your best interest to notify your employer of your diagnosis. If you are covered under your employer's health insurance plan, the company will notice a sharp increase in benefits paid out and you need to prepare everyone for that. Also, you will be taking time off on a regular basis for tests and doctor's visits, and you will need your employer's cooperation. I discuss notifying your employer in more detail in Week 2.

How much you tell your friends will depend on the type of relationship you have with them. If they are very close friends, you probably will eventually want to tell them everything. Their support will become more important to you as time goes by. They may react less emotionally than either your partner or your parents, and, if you are experiencing smothering or judgmental attitudes on the part of your partner and parents, you may find your friends' support appealing in contrast. And, unlike your parents and partner, your friends may be less likely to harbor anger.

However, there is really no reason to tell strangers about your illness. If you find yourself telling the TV repairman or the letter carrier about your condition, then you may be more anxious than you realize, an indication that you could benefit from sessions with a therapist.

Can I give cirrhosis to other people?

Absolutely not. However, if your cirrhosis was caused by hepatitis B or C, there is a possibility that you could give the virus to other people through unprotected sex or by using someone's toothbrush or by openmouthed kissing or by being careless with open cuts or abrasions. Even then, you are not at risk for passing on your cirrhosis, only the virus that causes hepatitis.

Sadly, you may discover, once you've made the choice to disclose your condition, that other people are fearful of contracting cirrhosis from you. They may tell you outright that they have concerns, or you may deduce it from the way they behave around you. You might feel that it is none of their business, and you're probably right. However, in these cases, I've found the best way to handle the situation is to volunteer information. Just assume that your friends, acquaintances, and relatives will fear the worst—namely, that your cirrhosis was caused by IV drug use or hepatitis or alcohol consumption. If none of those causes of cirrhosis apply to you, tell the people around you. Don't force them to guess. If any of the above causes do apply to you, be honest.

If your cirrhosis was caused by hepatitis, encourage the people around you to talk to their doctors about whether they need to be concerned about getting the disease from you or whether they should be vaccinated. If your cirrhosis was caused by IV drug use or alcohol consumption—and you have sought treatment for your addiction—then let the people you care about know the truth. Chances are they'll appreciate your honesty and react in a positive, supportive way.

IN A SENTENCE:

Use good judgment in talking about your illness by dispensing information on a need-to-know basis.

living

What Should I Be Eating?

IN MANY respects, diet is the key to longevity for cirrhosis patients. What a patient eats and drinks has everything to do with how long he or she will live. Different food considerations are needed at different stages of the disease.

If you have been diagnosed with cirrhosis at a very early stage, your doctor has probably told you to eat whatever you like, as long as it is healthy. By "healthy," I mean a diet that avoids potentially dangerous foods. The salt and fat content of foods may become concerns at later stages, but in the beginning your doctor will want you to avoid extremes in order to get a better idea of how your body is reacting to your cirrhosis.

On a daily basis, a healthy liver balances all the nutrients that enter the body. Proteins, carbohydrates, vitamins, minerals, fats—all have roles to play in your growth and development, and all are welcomed by the liver, which performs its functions like a circus juggler, balancing each nutrient with the other.

Problems arise when the liver is damaged and can no longer balance the nutrients entering your body. If you need a visual, think of the healthy liver as a two-handed juggler and an injured liver as a one-handed juggler. It's possible to juggle a couple of items with one hand, but the lowered efficiency level is apparent by the frequency with which third and fourth items hit the floor with a thud.

If diet is so important, you may wonder, why did you leave your doctor's office without a recommended diet? Doctors are not dietitians, and since a liver patient's dietary needs are determined by how well their liver is functioning, that can vary greatly from patient to patient, and from year to year. Unfortunately, there is no "one size fits all" diet for cirrhosis patients. Whether your doctor puts you on a special diet will depend on whether you experience complications from the disease. Depending on the severity of the complications, you may be placed on a low-fat, low-protein, or reduced-salt diet. If you are experiencing no complications, your doctor will be reluctant to make any adjustments to your diet.

What foods should I avoid?

Your first concern should be to eat no foods that will do you harm. Once you identify those foods and eliminate them from your diet, it will be easier to pursue a more proactive approach to what you eat so that you can benefit from your food choices.

There are two different categories of foods to avoid: (1) those that are vehicles for the transmission of infections, and (2) those with additives such as preservatives.

FOODS THAT MAY CARRY MICROBES

At the top of your list of foods to avoid should be any type of uncooked shellfish—oysters, clams, shrimp, or scallops. They carry a bacterium called *vibrio vulnificus*, which is known to be devastating to the human liver. The bacterium occurs naturally in seawater and is absorbed by shellfish. *Vibrio vulnificus* is the leading cause of seafood-related fatalities in the United States, causing 83 percent of all deaths attributed to seafood. The bacterium is so potent that 69 percent of the cases reported in humans are fishermen, oyster shuckers, or shrimpers who handled the shellfish while bringing them to market. The other deaths are attributed to unsuspecting individuals who ate infected shellfish without cooking them thoroughly.

Symptoms from this bacteria include vomiting, diarrhea, and abdominal pain, and once in the bloodstream of a person with liver disease, it can be fatal. Under no circumstances should cirrhosis patients eat raw oysters or clams. Clams, shrimp, and scallops are all right to eat if they have been thoroughly cooked.

Other foods that often carry viruses and bacteria include strawberries, lettuce, green onions, watermelon, and cantaloupe. Whether you avoid these foods will depend on whether you have been vaccinated for hepatitis A or whether you have complications of cirrhosis that make you more susceptible to infections. If you have not been vaccinated for hepatitis A, my advice is to avoid all of these foods uncooked until you have received your vaccination. If you have been vaccinated, they should be safe raw if carefully washed. Generally speaking, you should avoid salad bars where the food has been sitting for a long time and may not have been carefully washed.

FOODS WITH ADDITIVES

You should avoid all foods with nitrites or nitrates. They are mainly found in processed meats of the type usually sold in delis—pepperoni, salami, sliced turkey, sliced beef, etc. They can be dangerous because your body converts them into nitrosamines, chemical compounds that are known to be carcinogenic or toxic to the liver. In addition, if you eat processed meat and wash it down with iced tea, the combination of nitrites from the meat and tannic acid from the iced tea will create a potent carcinogen. With liver cancer a concern, that is exactly the type of chemical cocktail that a cirrhosis patient needs to avoid.

Match your diet to your symptoms. if you are experiencing ascites, you should talk to your doctor about how to reduce the amount of salt in your diet. The body requires up to 400 milligrams (mg) of salt per day for healthy functioning. Anything above that can be harmful to a person who has cirrhosis with ascites, but experts disagree about how far above that level it is safe to go. Dr. Carol Semrad, director of clinical nutrition at Columbia University, feels it is safe for a person with ascites to consume up to 2 grams of salt each day. "A good guideline is to restrict down to what we call a 2-gram-salt diet," she says. "If you just add no salt to your food, that's considered a 4-gram-salt diet, and then if you don't cook with salt and you eliminate salty foods and you don't put any salt on your foods, that's about equivalent to a 2-gram-salt diet."

If that is your situation, you should first stop adding table salt to your food. You also should stop eating canned foods, since they add salt as a preservative and for flavor. Avoid eating at fast-food restaurants, and pay strict attention to all over-the-counter remedies that you use (for example, two tablets of Alka-Seltzer exceeds the daily salt minimum). Red meat and fish should be avoided since they have a high salt content. Other foods with high salt content are soy sauce, canned soup, anchovies, corn, and ketchup. If you have ascites, a vegetarian diet can be beneficial.

If you are showing symptoms of sleepiness or confusion (encephalopathy), you should talk to your doctor about how to reduce the protein in your diet. The foods that contain the most protein are red meat, fish, pork, and poultry. The foods that contain the least protein are rice, eggs, broccoli, bread, milk, and spaghetti. A vegetarian diet offers the most potential for reduced protein and offers protection against encephalopathy since vegetables produce less ammonia than do meat products.

If your iron levels are too high, you should avoid iron-rich foods such as liver, red meat, or iron-fortified cereals. Iron-rich vegetables such as spinach and turnip greens are not as threatening as the iron found in animal foods, since they are not absorbed as well into the body. Odd as this may sound, you also should avoid cooking in iron cookware since the food cooked in such cookware can absorb the iron.

Excess iron had been associated with liver cancer and liver failure. If you have cirrhosis, it is thought that even a normal amount of iron could cause additional damage. As a cirrhosis patient, the amount of scarring you have is directly related to the amount of iron in your liver. For that reason, you should treat iron as a potential poison.

10 Commandments for a Healthy Diet

DON'T:

1. Eat raw shellfish (oysters, clams).

2. Drink alcohol.

3. Eat processed meats.

4. Eat restaurant food that is not delivered hot on the plate (due to bacteria risk).

5. Eat while under stress (no arguments before, during, or after meals).

DO:

1. Divide your food intake into several small meals.

2. Drink plenty of water (unless you have ascites).

3. Sip fluids with your meals (fluids dilute your digestive juices, so you want to drink sparingly during meals).

4. Eat plenty of fruit (be sure to wash it first).

5. Avoid excess iron consumption.

If you are obese

If you are obese, you should work with a dietitian to formulate the right diet for you. The challenge for you is to lose weight while eating only the foods that are advisable for this condition. Stay away from fad diets—a diet that contains massive amounts of animal protein, for example, may help you lose weight, but the levels of protein that the diet recommends may further damage your liver.

My suggestion is to work with a qualified dietitian and then run the finished plan past your doctor for comment. Your dietary options will depend on whether you have complications from cirrhosis. For more on obesity and cirrhosis, see page 134.

IN A SENTENCE:

> *Your recovery depends on your ability to maintain a proper diet.*

learning

What You Need to Know about Hepatitis

ONE OF the things that makes hepatitis such an insidious disease is the stealthy approach it takes when it invades your body. It is a secretive disease that wears many masks and disguises, and when it visits it often does so without announcing its arrival.

The word *hepatitis* means "inflammation of the liver." You know what an inflamed throat feels like. It hurts and feels sore, and when you examine it you see reddish tissue that looks angry. An inflamed liver is a lot like a sore throat, except the inflammation is not where you can see it and it does not feel sore because your liver does not have cells with the same sensitivity as the skin cells in your throat.

For those reasons, your liver can come under vicious attack without the slightest outward indication that anything is wrong. The inflammation caused by the hepatitis virus can follow one of three routes—acute, chronic, or fulminant.

Hepatitis is classified as *acute* when the liver's inflammation lasts less than six months. Patients with acute hepatitis can be severely ill, but then make a complete recovery. It is classified as *chronic* when the inflammation lasts longer than six months.

And it is classified as fulminant when liver failure occurs within two weeks of the appearance of outward symptoms such as jaundice.

Since hepatitis is caused by a strain of viral microorganism, each of which is different, it is possible to classify each type according to the characteristics of the various viruses that are identified with each strain of the disease. Thus we have hepatitis A, B, C, D, and E, which may be further described as acute, chronic, or fulminant. Although all types of hepatitis can present an acute phase, hepatitis A and E are never chronic, and hepatitis C is almost never fulminant.

Hepatitis A

Sometimes called infectious hepatitis, it is the most common cause of acute viral hepatitis in the United States. Nearly 150,000 people a year in the United States are infected by the disease, and researchers estimate that one out of three people in the United States has been infected at some point in their life.

Hepatitis A is considered the least serious of the hepatitis viruses. Usually patients recover fully within six months. Since the liver repairs the short-term damage done by the virus without experiencing any permanent damage, the disease is not generally associated with either cirrhosis or liver cancer. Although several hundred people a year in the United States die of complications associated with hepatitis A, those situations usually involve overlap with other life-threatening diseases, such as hepatitis B or C—and in most instances the patients are over fifty years of age. Hepatitis A should be of concern to anyone who has been diagnosed with cirrhosis, especially if they are over fifty.

Hepatitis A is most commonly transmitted through food that has been contaminated by an infected individual who handles food, beverages, ice, etc., without properly washing his hands after a bowel movement. In those instances, the virus passes from minute particles of fecal matter into the mouth of an unsuspecting person and passes from the stomach to the small intestine to the liver.

Apart from fecal-to-mouth transmission caused by unsanitary food handlers, the virus can be transmitted in uncooked or undercooked foods such as strawberries, salads, and pastries. Sexual transmission of the disease has been associated with oral-anal sex and oral sex.

Individuals who are at increased risk of getting hepatitis A include:

O People who eat undercooked or uncooked restaurant or vendor food. I don't eat salads, fruit, or uncooked pastries from fast-food restaurants because the high employee turnover rate makes it difficult for managers to maintain effective hygiene control. The person who tossed your salad or sliced your fruit may have forgotten to wash his hands after a bowel movement and he may have forgotten to wear plastic gloves while preparing your food.

O People who have oral-anal sex.

O Men who have sex with men.

O People who travel in developing countries.

O People who work around sewage.

O People who spend time around young children. Due to inadequate hygiene habits, young children are common transmitters of hepatitis A, especially if they attend day care centers. Often children harbor the disease without ever displaying any symptoms, and adults can get the disease from them without ever making the association.

Symptoms of hepatitis A vary greatly. Some people have the disease without ever knowing it. Others display minor flulike symptoms. Symptoms of a more virulent case include abdominal pain, diarrhea, vomiting, and a sudden fever. Adults typically ignore those symptoms unless they develop jaundice or dark urine or itching.

The disease can be debilitating in serious cases and can make the patient ill enough to require hospitalization. In those instances, it is not unusual for patients to lose a month or more from work. In rare cases, the disease can quickly progress to fulminant status and require an immediate liver transplant.

The only certain way to diagnose hepatitis A is with a blood test.

Hepatitis B

Hepatitis B was originally called serum hepatitis. The single greatest cause of cirrhosis, it has infected an estimated two billion people worldwide, killing one million people each year. Unlike hepatitis A, this strain of the disease cannot be transmitted through food. It can only be passed through blood, through sexual contact, or from mother to child during pregnancy. Of those who have the hepatitis B virus in their blood, only a small percentage are infectious and capable of giving it to others.

Prior to 1975, blood transfusions were a common means of transmission. However, since then, the U.S. blood supply has been screened for hepatitis B and that type of transmission is now rare. More common means of transmission through blood include the sharing of toothbrushes or nail clippers, tattoos and body piercing, intravenous drug use, shared straws used to snort cocaine, cuts from barbers or manicurists, open wounds, needle pricks in the health-care profession, and paper money that has been placed in the mouth. Hepatitis B can remain contagious for up to one week on paper or other surfaces.

Researchers have found that the hepatitis B virus is a hundred times easier to transmit sexually than the HIV virus. It can be passed through semen, vaginal secretions, or saliva. It cannot be passed on by dry kissing on the lips, but it can be passed on by oral-genital contact or any type of anal sex. There is no proof of deep-kissing transmission, but it is certainly possible, since the virus has been detected in saliva. Of course, the more sexual partners you have, the greater your risk of contracting the disease. Men who have unprotected sex with men are fifteen times more likely to get the disease than heterosexuals.

Transmission of hepatitis B to a child through childbirth is common in Asian and African countries, but it is becoming increasingly rare in the United States, where all pregnant women are screened for the virus. Today infants are routinely vaccinated against the virus, regardless of whether the mother tests positive for the disease.

Since there are three types of hepatitis B—acute, chronic, and fulminant—symptoms can vary. People with acute or chronic hepatitis B often don't know they have the disease; nor do they realize they can pass it on to others. Early on, the only symptom may be a vague sense of fatigue or weakness. Your liver may be slightly swollen, but unless a doctor examines you and discovers the swelling, your condition will probably go unnoticed until it progresses to cirrhosis, which could take ten, twenty, or thirty years. However, if you are jaundiced when you see a doctor, she will probably order a round of blood tests to get a reading on your **transaminases** (liver enzymes). If you have acute hepatitis B, your enzyme readings will remain high for about six months and then subside. If your readings remain high past six months, that increases the likelihood that an acute condition has progressed to a chronic state.

If your cirrhosis is the result of hepatitis B, it was probably acute at some point, but then progressed to a chronic condition. If you have been diagnosed with cirrhosis, you can likely rule out fulminant hepatitis B because it is so virulent that 85 percent of the people who have it die within a short time without a liver transplant.

Hepatitis C

An estimated one-fourth to one-third of people infected with hepatitis C have no idea that they are ill. That is one of the most insidious aspects of the disease, since it allows the disease to progress year to year until it eventually gets to a point where doctors have few options to treat it.

The Centers for Disease Control attributes about ten thousand deaths a year to hepatitis C, a statistic that invites labels such as "the silent killer" or "the silent epidemic." Hepatitis C is so pervasive that if you have been diagnosed with cirrhosis or liver cancer, the odds are that you have the hepatitis C virus in your body.

There are many ways to get hepatitis C, but the most common is through blood-to-blood transmission through intravenous drug use or blood transfusions. Some studies have suggested that intravenous drug use accounts for up to 60 percent of new hepatitis C infections. Patients are sometimes shocked to learn that a single experimentation with intravenous drug use twenty-five or thirty years ago was probably responsible for their infection. Other methods of transmission include tattooing and body piercing, childbirth, and through the sharing of household items such as toothbrushes or razors.

It is possible but not very likely to get hepatitis C through sexual contact, unless intercourse takes place while the woman is having her period or unless there are breaks in the skin of the mouth, penis, or vagina at a point where bodily fluids are exchanged. Rough sex, especially if it involves anal intercourse, offers possibilities for the transmission of the disease, which puts homosexual men at greater risk.

When symptoms of hepatitis C appear, they are identical to those of other types of the disease, but most people never display symptoms of any kind. If symptoms do appear, they are usually so mild—fatigue, decreased appetite, etc.—that they are attributed to the flu or minor stomach upsets. Most of the time a physical examination of a person with hepatitis C will uncover no abnormalities. Sometimes a physical examination will reveal an enlarged liver, but that doesn't occur often. Most of the time a person will have the disease for many years before it is detected. The only way to diagnose hepatitis C is through a blood test.

People who report symptoms such as jaundice are more likely to have acute hepatitis C. Ironically, individuals with hepatitis C who report the most symptoms are the most likely to see the complete disappearance of the disease from their system. It is the chronic strain of the disease that is most likely to lead to cirrhosis.

> *I was stunned when my doctor told me*
> *that I have hepatitis C. I feel great and I*
> *haven't had so much as a cold in the past*
> *five years. I thought I was in perfect health,*
> *but it turns out that I have a virus that is*
> *quietly chewing away at my liver.*
>
> —THOMAS A.

There are tests that can detect the hepatitis C antibody, but there is no vaccination for the disease. The prognosis depends on the person's age, gender, race, immune status, and genetic makeup. Women tend to develop cirrhosis from the disease less often than men. African-Americans have a higher incidence of the disease than Caucasians and they are less likely to respond to current treatment; in addition, African-American males are more likely to progress to chronic disease than Caucasians.

The younger a person is when they become infected, the slower the disease is likely to progress. In other words, it is better to be infected in your twenties or thirties than in your forties or fifties. Researchers have found that some people have a genetic makeup that allows them to avoid the most serious complications of the disease, while others have a genetic makeup that makes them more susceptible to serious complications.

The final variable is the immune system. Some people have immune systems that are effective at retarding the progress of the disease, while others have immune systems that seem to invite a rapid escalation of damage to the liver.

Hepatitis C is unpredictable in its progression. It is estimated that up to 85 percent of people who are infected with the virus will develop chronic hepatitis C, but doctors are unable to predict with any accuracy what percentage of chronic cases will turn into cirrhosis. Some patients develop cirrhosis rapidly after exposure. Some patients take years to develop cirrhosis. And some patients never develop cirrhosis.

Hepatitis D

Hepatitis D, which was not discovered until 1977, is sometimes called the delta gent or HDV. What makes it different is its tendency to coexist with hepatitis B or hepatitis C strains, since it cannot replicate on its own. However, it is a dangerous strain of the disease because it tends to worsen the B or C strain. Seventy-five percent of people diagnosed with hepatitis D can expect to develop cirrhosis.

Since hepatitis D is chiefly linked to hepatitis B, its prevention is dependent upon avoiding the B strain. It is spread in the same way—through infected blood—and it targets the same high-risk groups—intravenous drug users and homosexual men. There is no vaccine available for hepatitis D, but if you are vaccinated against hepatitis B, you are protected against hepatitis D.

The incidence of hepatitis D in the United States is currently low, but that could change as more troops return home from the Middle East, where the incidence is high. Theoretically, a soldier who is vaccinated for hepatitis B is protected from acquiring the D strain, but there is no vaccination for the C strain. Those cases may not be diagnosed for another twenty or thirty years.

Often the first indication that a patient has hepatitis D is complete liver failure, or mental changes that can range from mild confusion to coma, the result of toxins that affect the brain. The only effective treatment at that point is a liver transplant.

Hepatitis E

Hepatitis E is usually transmitted by water. The disease is rare in the United States and it is most often reported in India, Africa, Pakistan, Asia, and Mexico. It mostly attacks people aged fifteen to forty and it has a high fatality rate among pregnant women. The best way to protect yourself is to be careful what you eat and drink. There is no effective treatment for hepatitis E. Most people either recover fully without treatment or the disease progresses to fulminant hepatic failure, in which case it will prove fatal without a liver transplant.

IN A SENTENCE:

If your cirrhosis was not caused by hepatitis, you must be diligent in protecting yourself from the disease, since it could prove fatal on top of your existing cirrhosis.

Taking Your Vitamins

AFTER I was told I had cirrhosis, I was a little surprised that the only prescription I was given initially was not even written out on a prescription pad. "I'd like you to take multivitamins without iron," said Dr. Hall, my gastroenterologist. Subsequently, his advice was expanded by Dr. Regenstein, my hepatologist, who suggested I take the following supplements:

- ◯ Vitamin E
- ◯ Lecithin
- ◯ Folic acid
- ◯ Calcium
- ◯ Magnesium (if needed for muscle cramps)

Since no doctor had told me I needed vitamin supplements since I was a child, I was naturally curious about the role that vitamins play in liver disease, so I did a little research on the subject and learned that what I considered a childhood medication was essential to my survival as a cirrhosis patient.

As we've learned, the liver is the organ that processes and stores vitamins and minerals for future use. For example, a healthy liver may contain a two years' supply of vitamin A. Other vitamins have different "expiration" dates, but all are warehoused in fatty solutions maintained by the liver. A liver that has been damaged by cirrhosis cannot produce the fats necessary to store the vitamins, which means that they pass through the system without being used.

Healthy individuals can take a long-range view of their vitamin intake, because their livers will store the excess. However, since that storage does not happen with a cirrhosis patient's liver, it is essential that necessary vitamins and minerals be ingested on a daily basis. That is especially true of vitamin K, which is needed to make the blood clot. Bleeding problems are a symptom and a complication of cirrhosis, the body's reaction to an insufficient amount of vitamin K. Clotting problems occur when the liver does not have enough vitamin K to circulate in the bloodstream.

Multivitamins

The multivitamins without iron that I chose contained 3,000 international units (IU) of vitamin A, 60 milligrams (mg) of vitamin C, 400 IU of vitamin D, 30 IU of vitamin E, 1.5 mg of thiamin, 1.7 mg of riboflavin, 20 mg of niacin, 2 mg of vitamin B-6, 400 micrograms (mcg) of folic acid, 6 mcg of vitamin B-12, and 10 mg of pantothenic acid.

Vitamin A

Vitamin A belongs to a group of compounds called **retinoids** that are found naturally in egg yolks, liver, fortified milk, liver oil, margarine, and fish oil. In its plant form (**carotenoids**), it can be found in carrots, cantaloupes, sweet potatoes, and leafy green vegetables such as spinach or turnip greens. An important vitamin, A is needed to help keep the immune system healthy and to maintain normal vision.

For people *without* liver disease, the body's requirements are met in a well-balanced diet. It is unwise for a healthy person who eats well to take vitamin A as a supplement since high levels of the vitamin can cause cirrhosis.

For people *with* liver disease, vitamin A is potentially toxic, especially when mixed with alcohol or acetaminophen (Tylenol). The recommended dose of vitamin A is 1,000 mcg for men and 800 mcg for women. Cirrhosis patients who mix alcohol or acetaminophen with that dosage—or higher—risk fatal complications.

If you drink or take acetaminophen on a frequent basis, you should never eat animal liver or cod liver oil. Vegetables that are high in vitamin A may be consumed freely, but cirrhosis patients should avoid juice drinks that contain large amounts of blended fruits and vegetables.

Vitamin B complex

This supplement consists of eight different vitamins, including thiamine (vitamin B-1), riboflavin (vitamin B-2), niacin (vitamin B-3), pantothenic acid (vitamin B-5), pyridoxine (vitamin B-6), cyanocobalamin (vitamin B-12), folate, and biotin. All are safe for cirrhosis patients, expect niacin, which can be harmful in large doses.

Thiamine. Needed for digestion, it can be found in whole-grain cereal, brown rice, pork, and soybeans. Cirrhosis patients often have a shortage of this vitamin, a condition made worse by caffeine. When that happens, hospitalization may be required.

Riboflavin. Needed for energy production and for the repair of organs, it can be found in milk, leafy green vegetables, and liver. When the body does not have enough riboflavin, sores will appear in the corner of the mouth and the vision may be affected. When the body ingests too much riboflavin, the urine will turn a bright yellow.

Niacin. Necessary for healthy skin, it can be found in peanuts, meat, vegetables, and eggs. High doses of this vitamin can be dangerous for cirrhosis patients. Sometimes niacin can cause the face, arms, and chest to flush bright red, a harmless condition not to be confused with the reddened palms typical of cirrhosis patients (palmar erythema).

Pantothenic acid. Needed to convert proteins, fats, and carbohydrates into energy, it can be found in nuts, meat, eggs, and fresh vegetables. It is sometimes called the "antistress" vitamin. Deficiencies of this vitamin are rare in healthy people but fairly common in alcoholics.

Pyridoxine. Needed for the metabolism of proteins, carbohydrates, and fats, it assists in the production of red blood cells and hormones. It is found in salmon, nuts, brown rice, and most meats. Large doses have been linked to nerve damage.

Cyanocobalamin. Needed for the manufacture of red blood cells, it can be found in milk, eggs, fish, and meat. Deficiencies occur in people who consume excess amounts of alcohol and in people with chronic liver disease who follow a vegetarian diet. Symptoms of a deficiency include rapid heart rate, fatigue, mood swings, and short-term memory loss. Sometimes severe psychosis can be associated with a cyanocobalamin deficiency. People who are taking proton pump inhibitors (Zantac, Tagamet, or Prilosec) to block stomach acid should be checked for a deficiency.

Folate (folic acid). Needed for good brain function, it can be found in oranges, brown rice, cheese, and whole grains. A deficiency is common in people with alcoholic liver disease and in women who take oral contraceptives. Symptoms of a deficiency include memory loss, a sore red tongue, and fatigue.

Biotin. Needed for healthy hair, skin, and nails, it can be found in milk, poultry, and brewer's yeast. Some doctors believe it is beneficial for patients with nonalcoholic fatty liver disease.

Vitamin C

Vitamin C is an antioxidant that is thought to be helpful in the production of **interferon**, which occurs naturally in the body. It can be found in most fresh fruits and vegetables. If your cirrhosis was caused by hepatitis C and your doctor is treating you with interferon, she may ask you to take vitamin C to supplement the interferon being produced by your body. If your cirrhosis was caused by something other than hepatitis C, your doctor probably won't recommend a vitamin C supplement unless you smoke cigarettes or use antidepressants.

Vitamin D

Vitamin D is important because it is essential to the absorption and metabolism of calcium. It can be found in fortified milk, egg yolks, cod liver oil, and most kinds of fish, but its most common source is sunlight. Healthy people need only fifteen minutes of sunlight several times a week to absorb the minimum requirements of vitamin D.

In her book *Hepatitis and Liver Disease*, Dr. Melissa Palmer recommends that people with cirrhosis supplement their diets with calcium and vitamin D, especially if they are taking **prednisone**. The U.S. government's recommended dose of vitamin D is 200 IU per day, but she recommends a daily dose of between 400 and 800 IU, provided levels of calcium in the blood and urine are monitored by a physician. She points out that excessive amounts of vitamin D can lead to dangerous deposits of calcium in the heart, kidneys, and blood vessels.

Vitamin E

Vitamin E is an antioxidant that protects red blood cells. It can be found in vegetable oils, nuts, dark leafy vegetables, and whole grains. The U.S. government recommends 100 IU of the vitamin each day, but a balanced diet usually supplies that amount. Higher doses of between 400 to 800 IU each day are recommended by physicians for individuals with liver disease, especially cirrhosis.

Some studies have suggested that vitamin E may slow the progression of liver disease and may be beneficial in the treatment of hepatitis C. Cirrhosis patients who are experiencing variceal bleeding should not take vitamin E unless it is prescribed by their physician. Cirrhosis patients taking the vitamin should discontinue its use for least a month before undergoing a biopsy or any other surgical procedure.

Vitamin K

Vitamin K is used in the manufacture of the protein prothrombin, which is necessary for proper blood clotting—without it you would hemorrhage from even the smallest cut. It is found in spinach and other leafy green vegetables, potatoes, liver, and cereal. Since half of the vitamin K used by the body is manufactured by bacteria that live in the intestines, a deficiency can occur if people abuse laxatives, antibiotics, or mineral oil for an extended period of time. If you have a vitamin K deficiency caused by something other than cirrhosis, your doctor may give you a vitamin K injection to correct the imbalance. However, if you have a deficiency that is caused by cirrhosis, an injection would be pointless since your liver would be too badly damaged to process the vitamin.

Lecithin

Lecithin is a fatty substance produced daily by the liver. Found naturally in peanuts, soybeans, wheat germ, and eggs, it is an essential building block for cell membranes, which harden when it is not present, and it acts as a shield around the brain to protect it. A ten-year study of baboons found that lecithin prevents severe liver scarring and cirrhosis, but no human studies have yet been completed. Other studies have suggested that lecithin supplements may prevent gallstones and assist in the treatment of liver problems caused by hepatitis.

Magnesium

Magnesium is the fourth most common mineral in the human body. It is needed for hundreds of biochemical reactions, but it primarily helps maintain healthy muscle and nerve function and supports the immune system. Green vegetables are a good source of the mineral, along with legumes, nuts, and seeds.

In times of stress, the liver needs increased amounts of magnesium to handle the metabolism that is necessary for magnesium-dependent enzymes. Without an adequate supply of magnesium in the system, the body becomes more susceptible to stress.

Symptoms of magnesium deficiency included muscle spasticity, loss of coordination, nausea, diarrhea, and tremor. Probably the best indication that you have a magnesium deficiency and need a supplement is muscle cramps. Most doctors recommend magnesium on an as-needed basis.

Calcium

Calcium is a mineral that is essential for blood clotting, muscle contraction, and healthy teeth and bones. Without it, bones would become weak and brittle—and they would be susceptible to osteoporosis. Since osteoporosis is associated with many liver diseases, it is important for cirrhosis patients to either eat food rich in the mineral or supplement their diet with it. Good natural sources of calcium include dairy products, canned sardines with bones, and tofu.

Vitamins and supplements have been a favorite topic for newspaper, magazine, and television features for many years and we witness a surge in stories each time a new study suggests health benefits for a specific vita-min or supplement. Usually, those "benefits" are later qualified or repudi-ated by additional studies. For that reason, it is sometimes tempting to undervalue the benefits of vitamins and supplements. However, cirrhosis is a disease for which the benefits of vitamins and supplements are well documented, and you should follow your doctor's recommendations by tak-ing the exact dosage that he or she prescribes for you.

IN A SENTENCE:

> *Take the vitamins your doctor has recommended daily to ensure your body gets the nutrients it needs.*

learning

Your Disease May Be Caused by Drug Reactions

I guess I'm just too trusting.
When my doctor told me I had diabetes
I was devastated. I took the medication
he prescribed, no questions asked, thinking my
condition was under control. Several weeks later I
learned that the medication had damaged my liver.
Now I'm waiting for a liver transplant.

—EVELYN G.

MANY PRESCRIPTION and over-the-counter drugs can cause hepatitis and unexplained liver-test elevations. When that happens, there may be no symptoms and the patient may go for years without knowing that his liver has been affected by the drugs.

The prevalence of drug-induced liver disease is one reason why an evaluation of a patient's medication history by a physician is an essential first step in the diagnosis process when a patient presents himself to the physician with symptoms of liver disease.

If the physician suspects a drug reaction, she may want you to discontinue taking the medication to determine if the abnormality will resolve itself. If that is the case, and restarting the medication is accompanied by a return of the abnormality, the physician will have convincing circumstantial evidence that your medication is the culprit.

The next step for the physician is to determine if further discontinuance of the medication will be helpful or harmful to you. For example, if your medication is preventative in nature, such as in controlling cholesterol, it is unlikely that your physician would consider the risk of continuing the medication worth keeping you on it.

On the other hand, if your medication is to control symptoms related to seizures or high blood pressure or psychosis, your physician may very well decide that it is riskier to take you off the medication than it is to keep you on it. However, before making the decision to leave you on the medication, your physician will want to run blood tests to assess your liver function. In some instances, the problems may be due to the use of a short-term medication. Most reactions occur within five to ninety days of exposure. In those cases, there is not much your doctor can do once the drug has been withdrawn from your system: your symptoms will either subside or they will escalate.

Sometimes drugs that normally do not cause problems will produce adverse reactions in some individuals. The anesthetic halothane is an example. It is considered statistically safe—it causes hepatitis in one in 10,000 cases—but for those few who react badly, statistical safety has little meaning. There is evidence that repeated exposure to halothane increases your risk of developing hepatitis, so even if you have had the anesthetic previously without ill effect, it may not be safe for you to use again. Fortunately, halothane is virtually never used anymore in the United States.

If you already have cirrhosis and you are scheduled for surgery, you may want to tell your anesthetist that you also have concerns about methoxyflurane and enflurane, two anesthetics that have been linked to liver damage.

There are many drugs on the market that can potentially cause liver damage, or, if you already have cirrhosis, speed up its progress and put you on a fast track to a liver transplant. That is not surprising, if you think about it, because it is the liver that is responsible for metabolizing each drug you take. For that reason, it is the most drug-sensitive organ in your body.

Drugs you should avoid

Since your survival as a cirrhosis patient may depend on the questions you ask your doctor, it is helpful to remember that the ultimate responsibility for your good health depends on your ability and willingness to educate yourself about the potential dangers you face from a variety of sources. All prescription and over-the-counter drugs should be scrutinized carefully and the risk/benefit should be assessed before the medication is ingested. If there is any question in your mind about its safety, you should avoid the drug until you can receive expert advice.

Advises Dr. Fredric Regenstein: "Any patient developing an unexplained ALT/AST elevation more than two to three times the upper limit of normal should be watched very closely or taken off medications they are taking that have been associated with liver damage."

What follows is a list of drugs that have the potential to cause serious damage to your liver. If you used any of these drugs prior to your diagnosis of cirrhosis, they have may played a role in your illness. If the drugs were prescribed to you after your diagnosis, you will want to ask your physician about the potential side effects of the drugs.

○ **Acetaminophen (Tylenol).** An over-the-counter pain medication that is popular because it does not cause the stomach problems that are common with aspirin, acetaminophen is a major cause of liver damage when taken in excessive quantities or when combined with alcohol. However, the drug is perfectly safe if you do not take more than 2,500 mg in a day (five extra-strength tablets) Many physicians recommend acetaminophen to liver patients in small doses because they consider it preferable to aspirin, which can cause serious bleeding problems. Besides Tylenol, other brand-name drugs that contain acetaminophen include Darvocet, Valadol, Valorin, Vicodin, Percocet, aspirin-free Excedrin, Comtrex, Lortab, Lorcet, Zydone, Norco, Esgic, and Aceta with codeine. (Acetaminophen is known as paracetamol in the United Kingdom.) One of the problems associated with acetaminophen is that it is in so many over-the-counter and prescription medications that it is easy for people to inadvertently overdose by taking the recommended doses of several different medications containing the drug.

○ **Acetylsalicylic acid (aspirin).** Since one of the functions of the liver is to regulate blood coagulation (clotting), one complication of cirrhosis is a tendency for excessive bleeding due to ineffective clotting mechanisms. Aspirin is a dangerous drug for cirrhosis patients since even in small doses it can cause bleeding in the gastrointestinal tract and cause kidney problems. One of the first things you should ask your physician once you have been diagnosed with cirrhosis is for a recommendation for pain medication. His or her choice will depend on how advanced your liver disease is. Dr. Sanjiv Chopra recommends that patients who cannot stop drinking, or who have bleeding problems due to liver disease, use heating pads or acupuncture instead of aspirin or Tylenol for the relief of chronic discomfort— or perhaps seek advice from a pain-management specialist. Aspirin is in a class of drugs called nonsteroidal anti-inflammatory medications (NSAIDs) that also includes Advil, Aleve, and Motrin.

○ **Diazepam (Valium).** This is a psychotropic drug, commonly called a tranquilizer or antianxiety medication, that is dangerous to cirrhotic patients because it can cause weakness, confusion, and falling. It is not significantly toxic to the liver.

○ **Coumadin.** This is an anticoagulant that is more commonly referred to as a blood thinner. It is not significantly toxic to the liver, but it is dangerous for people with cirrhosis because it can cause bleeding.

○ **Tetracycline.** This is an antibiotic that has been linked to fatty liver disease. It is especially dangerous for pregnant women during the last half of the pregnancy.

○ **Methotrexate.** This drug is commonly used to treat psoriasis and other rheumatic diseases. It has been shown to cause cirrhosis, but since it does so without affecting the enzymes measured in blood tests, the only way to gauge potential damage to the liver is through a liver biopsy.

○ **Oral contraceptives.** Since birth control pills have been linked to liver tumors, it may be safer to use an alternative method of birth control if you have been diagnosed with cirrhosis, hepatitis, or fatty liver disease.

○ **Ibuprofen (Motrin).** This pain reliever is rarely toxic to the liver, but it can lead to bleeding and fluid retention, or kidney problems, in patients with cirrhosis.

○ **Tamoxifen.** A breast cancer medication that causes acute hepatitis.

○ **Anabolic steroids.** A medication prescribed for muscle growth that is linked to liver tumors.

○ **Estrogens and testosterone.** As with oral contraceptives, these hormones have been linked to liver tumors.

○ **Isoniozid (INH).** A drug used for the treatment of tuberculosis. It should be used with caution in patients with preexisting liver disease.

○ **Diltiazem (Cardizem).** A blood pressure medication that has been linked to liver damage in dogs and rats and to jaundice in humans. However, it rarely causes human liver damage.

○ **HMG-CoA Reductase Inhibitors (Zocor, Lipitor, Lescol, Mevacor).** These are the so-called statin class of drugs used to lower cholesterol. They are among the most frequently prescribed drugs in the United States. Studies have shown that hepatitis occurs in about 1 percent of patients receiving starting doses and in about 2 percent of patients who receive maximum doses. However, for some people, the drugs can be lifesaving.

○ **Rosiglitazone (Avandia) and Pioglitazone (Actos).** These are drugs used to treat diabetes. They should be used with caution in patients with cirrhosis because they have a tendency to cause fluid retention. If you are taking these drugs and develop symptoms of liver problems, Dr. Howard J. Worman recommends that you discontinue the medication if your blood enzyme tests produce scores of more than 1.5 times normal. Ironically, these drugs appear to be beneficial for patients with liver disease due to NASH.

IN A SENTENCE:

> *Prescription and over-the-counter drugs are a common cause of liver disease and possibly cirrhosis, so be sure to inform your doctors and pharmacists of every medication you are taking.*

living

Taking Care of You

*Two days after I learned I had cirrhosis I
went to work and one of my coworkers was
upset because her boyfriend wanted to
go fishing with the guys.
I thought, "What a wonderful idea!"*

—SARAH G.

YOU'VE KNOWN that you have cirrhosis for a week now. You've balanced that life-altering knowledge with the obligations you have to others. You've tried to comfort loved ones as they've tried to comfort you. You've gone to work and done what was expected of you. If you have children, you've made their breakfast and gotten them off to school. You've done the dozens of things that it takes to get through the day.

What you probably haven't done is taken a "time out" to focus on yourself.

For the past six days, your mind has been reeling with thoughts and concerns about your long-term future. Now is a good time to make some short-term plans. Depending on your personality type, it may be a good time to take a few days, perhaps even an entire week, off from work for the sole purpose of doing something nice for yourself.

Take a vacation

Plan a fishing trip. Go antiquing—the type of outing that requires you to travel from town to town. Go visit that beloved relative you haven't seen in years. Visit a spa for a massage and some pampering. If you live alone and have a pet, take your pet and go to the beach—or rent a cabin in the mountains. If you are married, or if you are involved in a close relationship, explain to your significant other that your desire to go on a "solo trip" is nothing personal. You simply want to commune with nature and get in touch with your innermost feelings.

Stress is bad for your liver

Coping with stress is key to boosting the effectiveness of your medical treatment. One of the best ways to relieve your stress and separate yourself from life's little annoyances is to either take a vacation or schedule short breaks into your daily routine, even if it's only twenty minutes or an hour each day.

When Henry F. learned he had cirrhosis, he surprised all his friends by loading up his SUV with camping gear and heading out for a weekend in the mountains. His friends thought that he should spend that time with them, but his instincts were to get in touch with his feelings without the distractions and obligations of friendships.

Upon his return, he felt refreshed and better able to deal with the new stress in his life. In his case, one of his old stresses was a quarrelsome friend who took more out of the friendship than he contributed. To the friend's surprise, Henry told him he no longer wanted to be friends. Says Henry, "I was tired of fighting with him over every little thing—from x to y—and I'd always end up in a bad mood. I realized that now, I needed to put myself first."

If your goal is to have a normal life expectancy, you owe it to yourself to take charge of the stress levels in your life, even if it means changing the dynamics of long-standing relationships. The important thing for you to remember is that chronic stress has been shown to weaken the immune system.

From 1982 through 1992, psychologist Janice Kiecolt-Glaser and immunologist Ronald Glaser, both members of the faculty at the Ohio State University College of Medicine, conducted research that showed, among other things, that a student's immunity went down every year under the simple stress of the three-day exam period. The students who participated in the study had fewer of the cells needed to fight tumors and viral infections and they almost stopped producing immunity-boosting gamma interferon and infection-fighting T cells. Other researchers subsequently found that chronic stress can wear down the immune system.

I realized after my diagnosis that I no longer had a need for troublesome and argumentative friends, colleagues, store clerks, and others—and so I set them free. You might sit down and make a list of the things in your life that are causing you stress. Divide the list into groups of things that you cannot change and things that you *can* change. Some of the things on that list will relate to people. Other things will relate to social or business commitments you have made, or even repairs that need to be made around the house. Once you have your list, you should then make the hard decisions that your liver is counting on you to make. Be bold! Be decisive! Take charge of your life!

Embrace feelings of loneliness

*This may sound weird, but the thing that freaked
me out the most about being diagnosed
with cirrhosis was the way my wife
stared at me when she thought I wasn't looking.*

—EDWARD G.

You may feel like your loved ones are watching you for any change in your condition. They may project their own fears onto you. You may see the emotional wheels turning inside your spouse's head when he or she looks at you. Indeed, one of the most common questions for a cirrhosis patient to ask a loved one is, "Why are you looking at me like that?"

If you have good days, they will think you are being brave. If you have bad days, they will feel guilty, as if they are to blame. You don't need someone, even a loved one, to tell you how you feel about your illness. You need to discover that for yourself.

Sometimes a spouse will overreact and either smother you with attention or withdraw from you altogether. He or she may try to do everything for you, even to the point of pushing you aside, or may sit back and offer to do nothing for you.

The first few days after you receive your diagnosis, you may feel a profound sense of loneliness. That is because for perhaps the first time, you realize that ultimately, you cannot control what happens to your body—it functions apart from your will. Life is a mysterious journey that each of us makes. It is important for you to understand that it's natural to feel alone after receiving a serious diagnosis. This loneliness is temporary, and it is neither good nor bad, but a vehicle for exploring your inner self.

Loneliness is not the same thing as isolation—you can be surrounded by the most supportive friends and family and still feel lonely. Isolation is the process by which you shut others out; it is a closed door that prevents your growth. Loneliness is the door through which you enter an expanding life. You should embrace your loneliness because by doing so, you will you learn to love yourself.

There is an invisible part of yourself that exists apart from the physical self that is known to your friends and loved ones. Whether you call that part of yourself your mind or your soul matters little. What matters is that you understand that it exists and it is open to exploration. Loneliness, taken in small doses, can be a positive experience if you use it for self-awareness. The purpose of taking a few days off to spend time alone is to open the door on an essential truth: life is brief, and only through a fuller realization of self can you achieve a level of inner peace. You are the only person who can experience that realization, or even define it, since that process is different for each person.

One way to take charge of your illness is to meditate on the following: *Loneliness leads to inner peace, which leads to healing.*

IN A SENTENCE:

Take some time off to get to know yourself and alleviate stresses.

learning

Autoimmune Hepatitis

It was the best of times,
it was the worst of times.

—CHARLES DICKENS,
A Tale of Two Cities

DICKENS WAS referring to a specific time in history, but he might well have been describing the feelings of a liver patient who has just been diagnosed with autoimmune hepatitis. That is because autoimmune hepatitis is a disease that can either spiral out of control in a short period of time and require the patient to have a liver transplant, or it can respond to specific medications that put the disease into remission.

There is not much middle ground with this disease. It is either a cause for cautious celebration (considering all the other alternatives) or a cause for concern. Luckily, most cases fall in the former category and offer patients reason for optimism.

Despite its name, autoimmune hepatitis is not related to the viral diseases that are known as hepatitis A–E. The two diseases share a common name because their symptoms are almost identical. However, autoimmune hepatitis is not caused by a virus and cannot be transmitted to other people. The disease, as the name indicates, occurs when the body mistakenly identifies the liver as a foreign organism and attacks it with the immune system, causing cirrhosis.

There was a time when autoimmune hepatitis was called lupoid hepatitis because it was felt that it was related to lupus, but that name is no longer used. The two diseases are not related, but they do belong to the same category of autoimmune diseases as multiple sclerosis, psoriasis, rheumatic fever, Crohn's disease, rheumatoid arthritis, thyroid disorders, and ulcerative colitis.

No one knows what causes autoimmune hepatitis, but it is thought that some people may have a genetic predisposition to the disease and develop it after exposure to a virus such as hepatitis A or any number of prescription drugs, including Aldomet (a medication for high blood pressure) and nitrofurantoin, an antibacterial drug used to treat urinary tract infections.

Symptoms

Autoimmune hepatitis is a relatively rare chronic liver disease that affects fewer than 200,000 people a year in the United States. Approximately 80 to 90 percent of people with the disease are females between the ages of ten and sixty years. There is no explanation for why females are affected more often than males, but one theory has it that the gene that controls the immune system may be attached to the X chromosome. Since females have an XX chromosomal configuration, compared to the male XY configuration, it is believed this may increase their odds of getting autoimmune hepatitis.

As with some forms of viral hepatitis, patients often report no symptoms and learn that they have the disease after routine blood work reveals that their liver enzymes are above normal. In other instances, patients experience what appears to be an acute case of hepatitis, with severe inflammation of the liver.

Common early symptoms include fatigue, poor appetite, abdominal discomfort or pain, joint and muscle aches, and dark urine. If the early symptoms are not addressed, more serious complications may develop, including fluid retention around the stomach and ankles or bleeding in the esophagus or stomach. The severity of the complications is generally a good indication of the severity of the disease.

Diagnosis

Dr. Howard J. Worman of the Columbia University Medical Center feels that the disease should be suspected in any young patient with hepatitis, "especially those without risk factors for alcoholic, drug, metabolic, or viral etiologies." He points out that patients with one subtype of auto-immune hepatitis have serum gamma globulin concentrations more than twice normal and patients with another subtype may have normal or only slightly elevated serum gamma globulin concentrations, but they will have antibodies called anti-LKM (liver kidney microsome).

There is no one test used to diagnosis autoimmune hepatitis, but the major laboratory tools used to detect the disease are tests for ANA (antinuclear anti-body), SMA (smooth muscle antibody), and anti-LKM1 antibody. Also criti-cal are liver enzyme tests (in severe cases, the AST and ALT levels will be in the 400 to 800 IU/l (international units per liter) range and the bilirubin level may be around 10 mg; in milder cases the levels could be normal or close to normal) and a biopsy will show markers consistent with autoimmune hepati-tis, in addition to providing evidence of inflammation and cirrhosis.

Unlike viral hepatitis, which shows up as a specific virus in blood tests, autoimmune hepatitis is a more difficult disease to diagnose and depends on the physician's ability to assemble an assortment of unrelated conditions and indicators that sometimes resemble pieces of a complicated jigsaw puzzle. The International Autoimmune Hepatitis Scoring System for the Diagnosis of AIH offers the following guidelines to assist physicians with their diagnosis:

POSITIVE FACTORS	NEGATIVE FACTORS
Female gender	
High AST/ALT and low AP	High AP and low AST/ALT
High gamma globulin level	AMA positive
ANA, SMA, or anti-LKMAb positive	Positive for HBV or HCV
Negative for HBV and HCV	Positive drug history
Negative drug history	High alcohol consumption
Low alcohol consumption	Liver biopsy results inconsistent
Liver biopsy results consistent	
Concurrent autoimmune diseases in the patient or family	
Positive for relevant HLAs	
Positive treatment response	

Treatment

The good news about autoimmune hepatitis is that there is a specific treatment for the disease. Typically patients are given a combination of two medications: a steroid known as prednisone and an immunosuppressive drug called azathioprine (Imuran) that is often used to treat kidney transplant patients. Prednisone is usually effective without the second drug, but azathioprine combines with prednisone in such a way as to lower the dose, an important consideration in reducing the possibility of serious side effects.

The purpose of the drugs is to knock down the inflammation in the liver. If the inflammation can be stopped, it will stop the progress of the cirrhosis. In some cases the treatment has been known to actually reverse cirrhosis—if it is in its early stages. The idea is to start the patient out on doses strong enough to saturate the liver (prednisone, up to 60 mg daily; azathioprine, up to 100 mg daily) and then to gradually reduce the dosage to a point where it is less likely to cause complications.

Some patients report feeling better almost immediately after beginning the treatment. Remission usually occurs in 80 percent of the cases, although it sometimes takes one to two years for patients to reach that point. Half of the patients who go into remission remain in that state, while others require the medication for the rest of their lives. Patients who remain in remission have a normal life expectancy.

Complications of autoimmune hepatitis

The important thing to remember about the prednisone/azathioprine treatment is that it suppresses your immune system and makes you more susceptible to diseases of all types. That means that you should avoid people with infections of any type, especially children, since they may be carriers of hepatitis A in addition to the usual viruses.

While you are on the medication, you should be diligent in washing your hands on a regular basis and refrain from touching your eyes or the inside of your nose since those are primary ways of spreading infections. Since the medication will also reduce the number of blood cells needed for clotting, you should avoid situations where bruising or injury may occur.

It would also be wise to avoid fast-food restaurants, where your food is less likely to be handled by food preparers that wear gloves. If they handle your food after going to the bathroom, it will put you at risk for any number of viruses and bacteria, including hepatitis A. If you are not certain that you have immunity to hepatitis A, you should be cautious about eating any restaurant food that is not transferred to your plate with utensils.

Autoimmune hepatitis patients are not likely to experience the traditional complications of cirrhosis if the disease goes into remission. As a matter of fact, the most frightening complication of cirrhosis—liver cancer—may be less of a concern among autoimmune hepatitis patients. "I've noted that one complication of cirrhosis—primary liver cancer, or hepatoma [cancer that arises within the liver, not cancer that originates elsewhere in the body and then spreads to the liver]—is singularly absent in patients with autoimmune hepatitis," says Dr. Sanjiv Chopra. "In fact, I haven't seen a single case of this complication. A short while ago, when I gave a lecture on tumors of the liver at a Harvard postgraduate course, I polled an audience of approximately 400 U.S. gastroenterologists to see if anyone had seen primary liver cancer as a complication of autoimmune hepatitis. Not one individual in the audience raised his or her hand."

Other doctors have a different experience. "I hate to disagree with my friend and colleague Dr. Chopra, but I have seen a case of (liver cancer) in autoimmune hepatitis," says Dr. Fredric Regenstein. "It appears to be much less common than with some other types of cirrhosis."

For those rare patients who do not respond to treatment, the prognosis is not bleak by any means. There are other medications, such as cyclosporine A and tacrolimus, that have proven successful as immunosuppressants. Failing all other treatments, autoimmune hepatitis patients can take comfort in the fact that the five-year survival rate for patients who receive a liver transplant is greater than 80 to 90 percent, and the risk of recurrence of the disease in the new liver is extremely low.

IN A SENTENCE:

> *Cirrhosis caused by autoimmune hepatitis offers you good odds for long-term survival.*

FIRST-WEEK MILESTONE

What You Should Have Done by Now

O   YOU HAVE LEARNED THE BASIC
    INFORMATION ABOUT CIRRHOSIS.

O   YOU HAVE LEARNED WHAT QUESTIONS TO
    ASK YOUR DOCTOR.

O   YOU HAVE LEARNED WHAT BEHAVIOR YOU
    MUST CHANGE.

O   YOU HAVE STARTED YOUR VACCINATIONS
    FOR HEPATITIS A AND B.

O   YOU HAVE LEARNED WHAT DISEASES POSE
    A THREAT TO YOU.

O   YOU HAVE ELIMINATED ALCOHOL FROM
    YOUR DIET.

O   YOU HAVE LEARNED WHAT DRUGS TO
    AVOID.

Undergoing a Liver Biopsy

THE FINAL word on whether you have cirrhosis is the biopsy, a procedure that involves the removal, with a special needle, of a small piece of tissue from your liver. It is the last step in the diagnostic process and the only test that can definitively detect cirrhosis.

Unlike the heart or the lungs or the brain or the stomach and intestines, which can be examined by various machines, devices, and procedures that allow doctors to determine how they are working, the liver has only one test—the biopsy—that allows doctors to peer inside the organ. Even then, it provides information about only a small portion of the liver, usually enough to detect cirrhosis, but not always enough to pick up other serious diseases.

The biopsy is the ultimate diagnostic tool for liver disease, but because of the risks and expense involved, it is typically the last test your doctor will use to diagnosis your condition. Your doctor will not resort to this test unless the other tests suggest cirrhosis—or unless all of the other tests are inconclusive and he simply has a gut feeling that you have cirrhosis. A biopsy could come two weeks into your treatment or it could come three months into your treatment, depending on what your doctor suspects is the cause of your cirrhosis. Biopsies for suspected liver cancer are occasionally performed, but they are not routine since the needle used in the procedure could spread the cancerous tissue throughout the liver, depending on the location of the tumor.

Called a **percutaneous biopsy** because it involves penetrating the skin, the biopsy usually takes place in a hospital. About an hour before the procedure begins, you will be given a blood test to determine your platelet count and your prothrombin time. Platelets are the smallest blood cells involved in blood clotting and your prothrombin time is a measurement of how long it takes those cells to clot. If your platelet count is low or if your prothrombin time is elevated, the procedure may be postponed until your doctor can correct the situation with drug therapy. In the case of an elevated prothrombin time, a vitamin K injection may be all that is required.

This procedure will be performed while you are awake, but you may request a mild sedative. You will be asked to lie on your back with your shirt off, and an antiseptic solution will be applied to your rib cage at the location the doctor has chosen to access your liver. At that point a needle at the end of a syringe will be inserted and then withdrawn, a procedure that takes only about one second. Often the doctor will use a sonogram to find a clear path to the liver. During the process, a small piece of liver tissue will be sucked into the needle attached to the syringe. It is that tiny tissue sample that will enable a pathologist to determine if you have cirrhosis.

Biopsy is one of those words, like *autopsy*, that you hope will never be used in the same sentence with your name. The very thought of a liver biopsy is enough to invoke anxiety in most people—and I was no different. The thought of paying a stranger to insert a needle into my side and then withdraw it with enough liver tissue for a microscopic examination was far removed from my daily life experiences.

The procedure can be done on an outpatient basis, which takes some of the emotional sting out of it. *How bad can it be*, I wondered, *if they will let you walk out of the hospital a couple of hours after undergoing the procedure?* Well, the truth is that deaths from liver biopsies do occur, but they are rare in patients with normal platelet counts who do not show symptoms of advanced liver disease.

When I arrived at the hospital for the biopsy, blood was drawn so that a platelet count could be determined. One result of advanced liver disease is a low platelet count, which means that the blood experiences problems clotting. The doctors told me that my blood work was "excellent," which meant that they did not have to consider alternatives to a percutaneous biopsy.

One of the biggest anxieties I had—and which you may be feeling, too—was that the procedure would be painful. However, when I had my biopsy, I barely felt the needle. Others report little pain at the time, but say that they develop soreness in the rib area afterward. I did not.

Problems can occur during this procedure if the needle misses the liver and perforates another organ (especially the lung or intestine), in which case a blood transfusion might be necessary. In the event of a severe perforation, emergency surgery may have to be performed to stop the bleeding. Deaths from this procedure can occur, especially in patients with bleeding disorders, ascites, or elevated prothrombin times, but these are rare.

Once the procedure is completed, you will be held in the hospital for observation for about four hours so that your pulse and blood pressure can be checked and so that the possibility of bleeding problems can be eliminated as a concern.

The results of your biopsy

The material removed from your liver will be placed on slides and evaluated under a microscope by a pathologist. Like the ultrasound, the biopsy report is only as good as the pathologist who evaluates it. Sometimes pathologists see problems that don't exist. Sometimes they miss problems and report no abnormalities.

In my case, the pathologist who evaluated my biopsy correctly identified the cirrhosis, but missed the nuances of the liver tissue that indicated the possibility of an autoimmune disorder.

For chronic viral hepatitis patients, pathologists use a number of different scoring systems. Most of the systems use different grades and stages. Grades measure the amount of inflammation. Stages measure the fibrosis. A 4-stage system for fibrosis is among the most widely used scoring systems (stage 1 = mild, stage 2 = moderate, stage 3 = bridging, and stage 4 = cirrhosis).

This is the only test that will let you know for certain if you have cirrhosis.

The best advice I can give you about biopsy reports is to suggest that you ask for a second reading of the slides by a different doctor if your report is inconclusive, or if it is either "too good to be true" or suggests a need for radical therapy. In other words, don't make any major treatment decisions based solely on one reading of your biopsy.

IN A SENTENCE

> The biopsy is the most important test that you will undergo, so make certain that you understand the results.

learning

Interpreting Your Test Results

I keep taking all these tests,
but no one ever explains them to me.
It's all very frustrating

—WANDA P.

MOST OF the tests that your doctor orders for you will be entirely painless. The exceptions are the blood tests, which may sting when the needle is inserted into your arm, and the biopsy, which may cause you slight discomfort. For the most part, the worst thing about the tests is waiting for the results.

Interpreting the test results is your doctor's job, but it is important that you familiarize yourself with the tests in advance so that you can understand your doctor's analysis. When you return to your doctor's office after undergoing tests, the tendency is for the doctor to give you the analysis without explaining why the test results suggest one possibility over another. If you don't have enough background information on the tests to ask questions, you probably will sit quietly and contribute nothing to the discussion.

Be proactive when the time comes to look at your test results. Ask questions. Do not allow yourself to leave your doctor's office confused about any aspect of your test results.

Blood test results

If your blood work is within the normal range, your doctor probably won't provide you with any numbers. However, if one or more of tests exceed the normal range, your doctor will let you know. You probably won't be offered a copy of the test results, but if you request a copy it will be given to you.

LIVER ENZYME TEST RESULTS

O **Transaminases (AST and ALT):** The normal range for AST is 0 to 40 IU/l. The normal range for ALT is 0 to 45 IU/l. (IU/l stands for international units per liter and it is the most common measurement used.) Some doctors refer to the AST and ALT measurements as a "liver enzyme test" designed to measure liver function. However, it is not a liver function test, but rather a measurement of ongoing liver cell death or damage.

Usually AST and ALT readings are roughly equal. One exception is alcoholic hepatitis (AST readings are usually higher than ALT levels). These readings can range from 0 to the thousands (liver failure due to yellow fever will produce readings of 4,000 to 5,000). Any reading above 40 for AST and 45 for ALT will be of interest to your doctor.

The numbers will provide your doctor with clues about your condition, but not with a definitive diagnosis. Chronic hepatitis caused by a virus, drugs, or alcohol will usually give readings less than ten times normal (less than 450 for ALT and less than 400 for AST). Massive liver failure of the type that can be caused by shock or a massive overdose of toxic drugs can give readings several hundred times normal (4,000 to 5,000).

You would think that AST and ALT readings would be a clear indicator of cirrhosis, but that is not always the case. For example, patients who have had cirrhosis for a number of years can have readings in the normal range.

If your readings are high, your doctor will schedule you for additional tests. If your readings are normal, you may still be asked to undergo additional testing, especially if you display other symptoms of liver disease, such as jaundice, itching, etc.

○ **Alkaline phosphatase (AP) and gamma-glutamyltranspeptidase (GGTP):** These two chemicals are known as cholestatic liver enzymes. High levels are consistent with blockage or inflammation of the bile ducts. When bile fails to flow, it is known as cholestatic liver disease. GGTP is found mostly in the liver, but AP can be found in other organs, such as the intestines or the kidneys. Elevated levels of AP are indicative of liver disease only if the GGTP level is elevated as well.

Normal levels of AP range from 35 to 115 IU/l and normal levels of GGTP range from 3 to 60 IU/l. However, if your levels are higher than that, don't jump to conclusions. Cigarette smokers have higher AP and GGTP levels than nonsmokers. One alcoholic drink can affect your GGTP reading, as can a failure to observe a twelve-hour fast prior to having the blood drawn from your body.

High AP and GGTP levels can be caused by nonalcoholic fatty liver disease, liver tumors, gallstones, alcoholic liver disease, or drug-induced liver disease.

BILIRUBIN TEST RESULTS

Since this is a chemical that the liver produces itself when it processes dead or dying red blood cells, it is a good marker of the activity taking place inside the organ. It can be measured by blood tests or urinalysis. Normal levels are less than 1 mg/dl (milligram per deciliter). It is when bilirubin levels go up that your eyes and skin can turn yellow and your urine can turn a dark yellow, almost brown. Surprisingly, many people with liver disease never become yellow. And even when they do become yellow, it may be related to a cause other than liver disease.

Usually, elevated bilirubin levels are caused by viral hepatitis; tumors in the liver, bile ducts, or gallbladder; alcoholic hepatitis; primary biliary cirrhosis; and drug-induced liver disease. According to Dr. Howard J. Worman, the blood bilirubin concentration is usually normal until a significant amount of liver damage has occurred and cirrhosis is present: "The rise in blood bilirubin concentration is roughly proportional to the amount of liver dysfunction."

ALBUMIN TEST RESULTS

In patients with cirrhosis who have moderate or advanced liver dysfunction, the blood concentration of this protein may fall below normal levels. However, since other diseases involving the kidneys or intestines also can cause drops in the albumin level, a lowered level is not necessarily an indication of liver disease. The normal range for albumin is 3.6 to 5.0 g/dl.

PROTHROMBIN TIME (PT) TEST RESULTS

Since this is a measurement of how quickly your blood clots (coagulates), it will play an important role in whether you undergo a liver biopsy. If your coagulation time exceeds the normal range, your doctor will want to investigate the cause and prescribe medication that will bring it to within the normal range.

Since normal PT values can vary from lab to lab, a standardized rating system called the international normalized ratio (INR) was developed so that results from different labs could be compared. Your lab reports will show either the PT results or the INR results. The normal range for PT is ten to thirteen seconds. The normal range for INR is 1.0 to 1.4. If your test scores vary greatly from month to month, you might want to talk to your doctor about using the home test that was recently approved by the U.S. Food and Drug Administration. That way you can take more frequent tests and provide your doctor with a better idea of when and how often your score changes.

PLATELET COUNT TEST RESULTS

Platelets are the blood cells that help form clots. A platelet count is useful with patients who have cirrhosis or are thought to have cirrhosis. A normal platelet count is 150,000 to 450,000/microL x 10 to the third/microliter. A score lower than 150,000 x 10 to the third/microliter would indicate the possibility of cirrhosis, especially if the spleen is enlarged. Cirrhosis patients often have enlarged spleens because of the workload shunted to it from a damaged liver.

ALPHA-FETOPROTEIN (AFP) TEST RESULTS

This is the only test that your doctor can give you to determine if you are developing a specific liver tumor called primary hepatocellular carcinoma. A high AFP level will suggest the possibility of a tumor, but there are other reasons why you could have a high AFP level. What your doctor hopes to receive is a low AFP level, which will give him or her more confidence that you do not have a tumor. If your AFP level is high, your doctor will probably want you to undergo a sonogram or a CT scan.

HEPATITIS VIRAL SEROLOGICAL MARKERS TEST RESULTS

The test results will reveal whether you have hepatitis A, B, or C. If the tests are negative for all types of hepatitis, you doctor will be confident that your cirrhosis was not caused by that viral disease.

SONOGRAM (ULTRASOUND) RESULTS

The sonogram is usually the second test that your doctor will order. It won't help your doctor determine if you have cirrhosis, at least not directly, but it will help him rule out gallstones or tumors, both of which will be detected by the procedure. If your doctor tells you that the ultrasound found no abnormalities, you can probably rule out gallstones or tumors, but you cannot rule out cirrhosis since the ultrasound does not detect scar tissue. However, it will detect excess fluid around the liver and abdomen, one symptom of advanced cirrhosis.

Unlike blood tests, which are evaluated by objective measurements, ultrasounds are subjective in the sense that they are only as effective as the person who administers them. Radiologists read the photographic printouts from the exam, but the content in the printouts is totally dependent on the technician's skill with the equipment. The more thorough technicians will twist you into a pretzel if they think it will provide them with a better view of your liver.

Your doctor will show you the results of your sonogram if you ask to see them, but it is unlikely that you will understand what you are looking at because interpretation is an extremely specialized skill. However, to the trained observer, the sonogram will show blood flow through the liver; it will detect masses on the liver and estimate the size of the masses; it will detect the accumulation of fluids in your chest cavity; it will determine if your bile ducts are obstructed; and it will locate gallstones if they exist.

You will not receive a score as a result of your sonogram. Instead, your doctor will let you know if the images reveal any problem areas.

CT (OR CAT) SCAN RESULTS

Like the ultrasound, the CT scan is at its best when detecting tumors and gallstones. It is the best test available for imaging the liver and the surrounding organs, especially the stomach. However, when it comes to detecting cirrhosis or hepatitis or measuring the amount of scarring in the liver caused by cirrhosis, it is no better than the ultrasound. It can detect cirrhosis only if the disease is advanced enough to cause the liver to be shrunken and nodular.

If your CT scan reveals no abnormalities, your doctor will probably lose interest in it until such time as he has reason to think there is a possibility that you might have developed gallstones or liver cancer. If your doctor has reason to be concerned about either of those possibilities, she might ask you to undergo a second scan.

If the radiologist who evaluates your CT scan reports no abnormalities, remember that all that that means is that gallstones or tumors are not apparent. If your doctor suspects cirrhosis, she will want to move on to the next test.

LIVER-SPLEEN SCAN RESULTS

This test cannot diagnose cirrhosis in its early stages, but it can indicate cirrhosis if the scar tissue has significant buildup. If that is the case, the radioactive particles that were injected into your bloodstream will be absorbed by your bone marrow instead of your liver, and that will be evident in the scan. It also will indicate if the liver is shunting part of its workload to the spleen, in which case the spleen will be enlarged after having absorbed many of the radioactive particles that normally would remain in the liver.

ENDOSCOPIC EVALUATION

This is the test in which a lighted viewing instrument, commonly called an endoscope, is gently lowered down your throat, through your stomach, and into the upper part of your small intestine. Air will be pumped into the tube to inflate your intestinal tract, a procedure that will take the wrinkles out of your intestine and allow a doctor to view the openings of the bile and pancreatic ducts. A dye will be injected into those ducts through a small tube and X-rays will be taken to gather pictures. This procedure is not used to diagnose cirrhosis, but rather to identify other conditions that will be of interest in treating your cirrhosis.

The endoscope also can be used to look for enlarged veins (varices) in your esophagus, a complication of cirrhosis. At some point in your treatment your doctor will want to find out if you have varices and, if so, whether they pose an immediate threat. This is not an examination in which there are varying shades of gray: either you have visible varices or you do not.

YOUR CHILD-PUGH SCORE

As a culture, we like to receive a "grade" or a "score" when we take tests or compete against others. The same philosophy applies to cirrhosis patients. Most cirrhosis patients wonder how they compare to other cirrhosis patients. There is no direct way to do that on an individual basis—unfortunately, there is no World Series of cirrhosis—but there is a mechanism called the Child-Pugh score that can provide you with a numerical score that will not only let you know where you stand, statistically, compared with other cirrhosis patients, but will provide you with an estimate of your life expectancy. The test has five criteria: (1) total serum bilirubin; (2) serum albumin; (3) INR (your coagulation score); (4) ascites (fluid buildup); and (5) encephalopathy (indications of damage to your brain as the result of toxins not processed by your liver).

Here is how to determine your Child-Pugh score:

TOTAL SERUM BILIRUBIN
Bilirubin <2 mg/dl: 1 point
Bilirubin 2–3 mg/dl: 2 points
Bilirubin >3 mg/dl: 3 points

SERUM ALBUMIN
Albumin >3.5 g/dl: 1 point
Albumin 2.8–3.5 g/dl: 2 points
Albumin <2.8 g/dl: 3 points

INR
INR <1.70: 1 point
INR 1.71–2.20: 2 points
INT >2.20: 3 points

ASCITES
No evidence of ascites: 1 point
Ascites controlled with medicine: 2 points
Ascites poorly controlled: 3 points

ENCEPHALOPATHY
No encephalopathy: 1 point
Encephalopathy controlled with medicine: 2 points
Encephalopathy poorly controlled: 3 points

How to Interpret Your Score:

5 to 6 points: Child class A: You have a life expectancy estimate of fifteen to twenty years.

7 to 9 points: Child class B: You should be evaluated for a liver transplant. If you undergo abdominal surgery, you have a 70 to 80 percent chance of surviving.

10 to 15 points: Child class C: You have a life expectancy estimate of one to three years.

As of this writing, I am a Child class A and a candidate for a liver transplant, primarily because I do not drink alcohol and have never engaged in substance abuse. However, my classification could jump to a class B or C if any of the following cause complications to develop:

O   Severe infection of any kind
O   Pneumonia
O   Appendicitis
O   Gallstone attack
O   Any accident that requires surgery
O   Severe food poisoning
O   Prednisone treatment stops working

As you can see, holding on to a class A status requires a proactive approach to your condition. You must follow all the rules for good health. And you must, at all times, be prepared for the unexpected.

IN A SENTENCE:

> *Simply stated, your test results determine your future: ask your doctor to explain your test results and what the significance is for your condition.*

living

Dealing with Addictions

*The toughest thing I had to do
was to quit drinking. I never thought I was
an alcoholic until I tried to stop.
It was the hardest thing I've ever tried to do.*

—EMILY W.

I HAVE never had an addiction of any kind, but I have friends who have struggled with addictions for years—and I have encountered addicts as a social worker. I cannot even imagine the stress involved for addicts who are diagnosed with cirrhosis. Dealing with the disease is bad enough, but if you add an addiction to the mix, it must seem, to the person involved, like an impossible situation to overcome.

Addiction is a pattern of behavior characterized by problem drinking and drug usage that affects an individual's ability to function as a productive member of society. It is marked by an inability to limit alcohol or drug usage, a physical dependence on the substance that results in sweating, nausea, and anxiety when withdrawal is attempted, and the need for increasing amounts of the substance in order to feel its effects.

Addiction affects the brain by distorting the senses, causing depression, and inducing an energized state known as being "high." Anytime the body receives chemicals from an outside source, the brain ceases manufacturing some of its own chemicals, such as dopamine and endorphins, which increases the brain's dependence on the outside source of chemicals. If the outside chemicals are stopped abruptly, the individual goes into withdrawal—a state in which the individual experiences irritability, sleeplessness, and occasionally seizures.

If you answer yes to one or more of the following questions, you should ask your doctor for a referral to someone who specializes in addiction problems:

○ Have you ever gotten into legal trouble as a result of using alcohol or drugs?

○ Have you ever lied to friends or family about your alcohol or drug use?

○ Have you ever used alcohol or drugs in the morning or at bedtime to steady your nerves?

○ Have you ever tried to cut back on your drinking or drug use and failed?

○ Do you ever feel annoyed when people ask you about your alcohol or drug use?

If you fall into this category, I don't have to tell you that your survival depends on your ability to escape an addiction that may have dominated your life for years. There is no margin for negotiation. You *can* win your fight against cirrhosis—but not if you are continuing to use alcohol, cocaine, heroin, or any other drug to which you are addicted. Either you face up to your drug problem, or you succumb to the disease. There is no middle ground.

Perhaps you have thought about getting help with your addiction for years, but kept postponing it because there didn't seem to be any urgency to stopping something that brought you so much pleasure (though considering the hell the substance put you through, the pleasure aspect is debatable). Perhaps you thought, *I can always quit one day*. Consider today the day to quit.

If you are an addict with cirrhosis, it is important that you seek help immediately. Depending on the drug with which you have a problem, you might start with Alcoholics Anonymous or Cocaine Anonymous or Narcotics Anonymous or the Center for Addictive Problems. Of course, these organizations can help only you if you have made up your mind that you need help.

I know people who have walked away from drugs and not looked back. If it is beyond your ability to stop cold turkey, it is important that you start reducing your intake of drugs immediately, before you ever meet with a twelve-step support group or a counselor. Do it on your own. Keep a record of when you take a drink or use cocaine or heroin or whatever happens to be your drug of choice.

Keeping a record is one of the most important things you can do. I have found addicts to be extremely forgetful. They use drugs four times within four hours and remember using only twice. You may find that a written record of your drug use provides you with a sobering reflection of your problem.

If you are into drug use too deeply to find your way out with twelve-step support groups or a counselor, then a rehab center may be your best hope for bringing your life under control. Just as beating cirrhosis requires a positive attitude, so does beating your dependency on drugs. If you need help, you can contact Narcotics Anonymous at 818-773-9999, and you can obtain additional information from their Web site at www.na.org.

What if you can't stop drinking?

Albert H. told his physician right away that he had a drinking problem. He explained that he had been an alcoholic since college and had tried to quit several times. The longest period he ever went without alcohol was four weeks.

The physician pulled no punches. "Treating your cirrhosis is a waste of my time if you don't stop drinking," he explained. "If you do stop drinking, the chances are good that your cirrhosis will not progress beyond its present stage."

"What if I can't stop?"

The physician shook his head. "In that case, you should start putting your affairs in order."

Albert went home and poured himself a stiff drink. As he sat in his favorite chair and surveyed his den—and the photographs of loved ones enjoying better days—he resolved to try one more time to quit drinking. That evening he went to Alcoholic Anonymous and gave it another try. "My name is Albert and I'm an alcoholic," he told the group. "This morning my doctor told me that I have cirrhosis."

Later, two men approached Albert and introduced themselves, explaining that they, too, had cirrhosis. Albert seemed surprised. "When was the last time you had a drink?" he asked one of the men.

The man smiled. "Three years, two months, and eighteen days," he answered. "And for my friend here, it's been almost five years."

Albert was encouraged. It was a first step, but one that showed promise.

If you are unable to stop drinking on your own, I urge you to seek professional help and/or a support group. Your prognosis will depend on your ability to successfully complete one of several treatment options available to you, such as the Alcoholics Anonymous Twelve-Step Program, or various inpatient and outpatient treatment programs that rely on professional counseling and medications to help control the symptoms of alcohol recovery.

There is no expense involved with Alcoholics Anonymous, but the inpatient programs can be cost prohibitive unless you have very good insurance or considerable savings. These programs offer supervised detoxification in a hospital setting. Typically, the program begins with a "detox" schedule that requires a physical exam and then moves on to bed rest, a balanced diet, and nursing care during the withdrawal period. Once the withdrawal period is over, the patient is put on a program that involves continued medical monitoring, nutritional therapy, and an education program about alcoholism. Finally, the patient is introduced to a twelve-step self-help program.

Less expensive are the outpatient treatment programs that combine counseling and drug therapy with the services of self-help groups such as Alcoholics Anonymous. The least expensive treatment option would be to combine Alcoholics Anonymous with personal counseling by a licensed social worker or psychologist who specializes in dependency issues.

Thirteen principles of effective drug abuse treatment

The following principles were developed by the National Institute on Alcohol Abuse and Alcoholism:

1. No single treatment is appropriate for all individuals.
2. Treatment needs to be readily available.

3. Effective treatment attends to multiple needs of the individual, not just his or her drug use.
4. At different times during treatment, a patient may develop a need for medical services, family therapy, vocational rehabilitation, and social and legal services.
5. Remaining in treatment for an adequate period of time is critical for treatment effectiveness.
6. Individual or group counseling and other behavioral therapies are critical components of effective treatment for addiction.
7. Medications are an important element of treatment for many patients, especially when combined with counseling and other behavioral therapies.
8. Addicted or drug-abusing individuals with coexisting mental disorders should have both disorders treated in an integrated way.
9. Medical detoxification is only the first stage of addiction treatment and by itself does little to change long-term drug use.
10. Treatment does not need to be voluntary to be effective.
11. Possible drug use during treatment must be monitored continuously.
12. Treatment programs should provide assessment for HIV/AIDS, hepatitis B and C, tuberculosis and other infectious diseases, and counseling to help patients modify or change behavior that places them or others at risk of infection.
13. Recovery from drug addiction can be a long-term process and frequently requires multiple episodes of treatment.

> *My doctor told me that my cirrhosis*
> *was caused by hepatitis C. He asked me*
> *if I used drugs and I lied and said no.*
> *Isn't it enough that I quit using drugs?*
> *Do I have to tell my doctor everything?*
>
> —SARAH K.

If you have an ongoing alcohol or drug abuse problem (it does not even have to be at the level of addiction), it is essential that you notify your physician, since none of the treatments that he or she prescribes will be effective if you continue to use alcohol and/or drugs. You may be able to deceive your physician for months, as your condition deteriorates, but should you require a liver transplant you will not be able to deceive the transplant evaluation team—and alcohol or drug abuse will disqualify you from receiving a new liver.

IN A SENTENCE:

> *Treating substance abuse and addiction now is essential to improving your cirrhosis prognosis.*

learning

Alcoholic Liver Disease

Water is the only drink for a wise man.
—HENRY DAVID THOREAU

FROM ANCIENT times, people have been aware of the dangers associated with excessive alcohol consumption, yet that awareness has done little to curtail the use of wine, beer, or whiskey. Studies have found that medical problems associated with alcohol consumption affect about 10 percent of the population and result in alcoholic liver disease in about a quarter of those affected.

Most people seem to think that they know how much alcohol is bad for them, but the truth is that there are so many variables involved in alcohol consumption that the only way to be certain that you are in no danger—*especially* if you've been diagnosed with cirrhosis—is to abstain from alcohol use entirely. Genetics plays an important role in the development of alcoholic liver disease, according to the experts. In her book, *Hepatitis and Liver Disease*, Dr. Melissa Palmer writes that the stereotypical person who "can drink anyone under the table" is more likely to develop liver disease than people who are more easily inebriated. In other words, the more outward tolerance your body shows for alcohol, the more likely you are to experience serious damage to your liver, especially cirrhosis—and vice versa: the less outward tolerance your body shows for alcohol, the more tolerance your liver shows for the substance.

If you are asked to bet money on who will live the longest—the person who can drink her friends under the table, or the person who is the stereotypical "cheap date" who can't hold her liquor—put your money on the latter and you will win every time.

How the liver processes alcohol

The liver is the body's first line of defense against the toxins contained in alcohol. Despite all the glitzy advertising that depicts alcohol as a sophisticated instrument of social discourse, it is essentially a poison that affects every major organ in the body.

It is the liver's job to metabolize, or break down, alcohol into chemicals that are less injurious to the body. It accomplishes that in one of two ways: (1) with the help of enzymes that transform alcohol into a harmless substance similar to vinegar, or (2) with the help of specialized enzymes that convert fat-soluble substances into water-soluble substances. Some individuals have a genetic deficiency for the enzyme that converts alcohol to a vinegarlike chemical; for those people, the skin often becomes red and warm after just a few sips of alcohol.

Liver damage occurs when one or both of those systems fail or when the liver is overwhelmed by an excessive amount of alcohol. Accompanying a breakdown in normal liver function because of alcohol ingestion are problems with bone marrow production, abnormal heart rhythms, pancreatitis, and changes in the nervous system that can alter brain function and contribute to the development of psychosis and short-term memory lapses.

Risk factors for developing alcoholic liver disease

For reasons not clearly understood, women are at greater risk than men of developing liver disease as a result of alcohol consumption and are more likely to die of cirrhosis. Those differences have been attributed to lower body weight among women and hormonal imbalances; studies have shown that women are less likely to seek help for alcoholism. No definitive explanation has yet been recognized.

Since body weight and gender play an important role in alcohol metabolism, researchers have been unable to determine a "one size fits all" level of safe alcohol consumption. Generally speaking, it is felt that the consumption of twenty grams of alcohol on a daily basis for five years is enough to put a person at significant risk of developing cirrhosis. Twenty grams of alcohol translates to roughly two and a half bottles of beer or glasses of wine, or nearly three ounces of distilled spirits such as whiskey or bourbon. For women, the at-risk amount is thought to be much smaller.

Some people never develop liver disease, no matter how much alcohol they consume. Genetics seems to be a determining factor in those instances.

Three stages of alcoholic liver disease

○ Alcoholic fatty liver. A condition that can develop within three days of excessive alcohol consumption, usually among so-called weekend drinkers. Typically there will be no symptoms and the patient will not be aware that he has the condition. However, a physical examination will usually reveal a liver that has been enlarged by fatty deposits. If alcohol is discontinued at this point, there are usually no long-term consequences.

○ Alcoholic hepatitis. An inflammation of the liver due to the toxic effects of alcohol. The symptoms can range from mild discomfort to a life-threatening condition involving bleeding and swelling of the stomach or legs. This condition shares many of the symptoms of hepatitis A-E, but since it is not a virus, the inflammation will normally be reversed if the patient stops drinking.

○ Alcoholic cirrhosis. The final stage in alcoholic liver disease.

Alcoholics with cirrhosis

Alcoholism is responsible for most cases of cirrhosis worldwide (with hepatitis C a close second). Some researchers estimate the alcoholism-related numbers to be as high as 75 to 80 percent of all cases reported. However, those numbers are lower in the United States, where hepatitis C has had a greater impact than in other countries.

For an alcoholic who has been diagnosed with cirrhosis, it's important to understand that there is no safe amount of alcohol that can be consumed with this condition. Up until the point where you start developing cirrhosis, any damage done to your liver by alcohol is potentially reversible. That is not the case once you have cirrhosis. From that point on, each drink you take only worsens your prognosis.

The only upside, if you want to call it that, to continued drinking by a person with cirrhosis is that those who continue to drink are less likely to develop liver cancer than those who abstain. Of course, one explanation for that may be that patients who continue to drink may die from accelerated cirrhosis development before they can develop liver cancer.

Unfortunately, that is not the explanation that is likely to be seized by the alcoholic who may rationalize continued drinking as a way to prevent liver cancer. Make no mistake—continued drinking is *far* more likely to be prematurely fatal. Once complications to alcoholic cirrhosis appear, the disease is irreversible.

IN A SENTENCE:

If you have cirrhosis, alcohol consumption is unsafe in any amount.

WEEK 4

Building a Support Network

This may sound strange, I know,
but for the first few weeks after my diagnosis
I felt like an alien from another planet,
especially when I was out in public.

—CHARLES Z.

IT IS probably safe to say that your diagnosis of cirrhosis arrived at a time in your life when you thought you had just about everything figured out: maybe not life itself, but all the routines, large and small, that get you through the day.

Then along comes that phrase—"You have cirrhosis"—and your world is turned upside down. The routines that you have spent a lifetime perfecting must all be reevaluated and, in many instances, radically changed.

○ You used to enjoy a cocktail when you got home from work, but now that's a thing of the past.
○ You used to love quick lunches at your favorite fast-food restaurant, but then you started eliminating food items that were touched by human hands or that may not be fully cooked.

○ You used to love it when your sister brought her preschool-age children over to visit, but now you find yourself worrying about what microbes may be adhering to their sticky little hands, and it's just not the fun it used to be.

○ If you are single, you used to love meeting new people. That first good-night kiss was always a thrill. But now you worry if that kiss is harboring an infection.

○ You used to be able to eat anything you wanted, but that is no longer the case. You've found that you've developed an intolerance for dairy. If you eat dinner with friends, you find yourself asking questions you never thought you would hear coming out of your mouth. "Did you put salt in that?" "Did you wash that fruit?"

○ You used to enjoy going to your boss's weekend barbecues, but now you feel intimidated.

○ You used to mow the lawn without thinking about the pollen in the air, but now you wear a mask so that you will not get your sinuses agitated and get an infection that would require antibiotics. The last time you did that, neighborhood children asked if you were trying to be like Michael Jackson.

Sometimes it may seem like no one understands what you are going through, other than your doctor—not your significant other, not your family, not your colleagues at work, not the window clerk at the nearest post office. That is a startling realization to make.

For the first time in your life, you may understand that it takes more than love to have peace of mind: it requires some element of commonality with others in the same position that you are in, people who know from experience what you are going through.

Support from your spouse

Janet was one of those women who had it all—a loving husband, two great children, a profession that gave her a sense of worth, supportive parents, and an attractiveness that always turned heads. When her doctor told her that she had cirrhosis, her first reaction was stunned disbelief. Not until she left the building and called her husband, Haley, on her cell phone, did the tears start flowing. He was supportive, but since he knew no more about the disease than she did, he really didn't know what to say.

"We'll get through this," he said.

"But what's at the other end?" she asked.

"It has to be something wonderful because you're so wonderful."

The words that had always worked in the past when Janet had had a bad day now seemed hollow and left her feeling oddly alone. *Did he even hear me?* she thought. She fought it, but she could not help but feel a tinge of resentment toward Haley. Later, when they were both at home, he held her and tried to comfort her, but with limited success. There were things she needed to hear, but she didn't know exactly what they were, only that Haley didn't seem to understand her needs.

When you reach out to your partner for emotional comfort, consider that he or she may be just as frightened and needy as you are. Accept their support for what it is—a loving gesture that is meant to wipe away your tears. So what if it doesn't work? Accept it in the spirit in which it is offered and then quietly move on to find the type of understanding that you really need to deal with your new priorities.

Support from family

Cirrhosis will not make an unsupportive family supportive; nor will it make a supportive family unsupportive. Your family will respond to your crisis in the same manner in which it has always responded to crises.

If you have been blessed with a loving family, you can probably count on unlimited support as you make your way through a maze of new challenges. However, if your family has a history of dysfunctional behavior during times of crisis, be prepared for more of the same—and do your best not to be affected by it.

The most realistic way of dealing with this issue is to make a list of your expectations. Writing them down will help you clarify your thoughts. What is it exactly that you hope to receive from your family? Do you want family members to hug you each time they see you and make a comforting reference to your disease? Or do you want them to refrain from demonstrating their affection or asking you questions about how you feel? Do you want them to bring you food? Do you want them to drive you to your medical appointments? Do you want them to spend more of their leisure time with you?

The best way to get what you want and need from your family is to ask them for specific things from your list. That will make your family feel better and allow you to have more realistic expectations.

Support from friends

When I told various friends about my diagnosis, the response was always the same: "That's horrible—let me know if there is anything I can do." And then, distance. One friend went with me to my first series of appointments, but then stopped offering to go. Another friend that I usually spoke to on a regular basis stopped calling and sort of faded away.

Soon I noticed a definite pattern of retreat. It took a while for me to figure out that not only did my friends feel uncertain how to react to my disease, it was also uncomfortable for them primarily because it made them come to terms with their own mortality. For many people, emotional retreat is a basic response to unpleasant situations.

I realized it was up to me to bring them around. That hardly seems fair, does it? After all, *you* are the person with a life-threatening disease. But you may have to reach out to your friends.

As with family members, the best way to get what you want and need from your friends is to ask them to help you with specific things, such as accompanying you to your doctor's office or to the hospital for tests. If you need someone to bring you dinner because you don't feel like preparing it, call a friend and ask for that specific favor.

Friends can be a terrific asset, but it is really up to you to communicate your needs to them. Just be specific when you let them know what you need.

Seeking out other cirrhosis patients

Family members and loved ones cannot always separate your needs from theirs in such a way as to be helpful to you. You might benefit more from the help of other patients who are going through what you are experiencing.

In Tennessee Williams's *A Streetcar Named Desire*, Blanche DuBois comments on her escorts to a mental hospital with the words, "Whoever you are—I have always depended on the kindness of strangers." Not only did Williams have a way with words, he had an uncanny knack for understanding the complicated needs of people in distress. Like Blanche DuBois, cirrhosis patients are often dependent on "the kindness of strangers."

If your cirrhosis was caused by alcohol abuse, you may already be acquainted with Alcoholics Anonymous. If not, you should get acquainted without delay. The organization is based on the principle that when it comes to addiction, strangers can often provide more comfort and guidance than loved ones.

Cirrhosis is not an addiction, but the principle is the same. What you need more than anything else at this point in your life is people who can talk to you about your disease from experience. Unfortunately, there are no comparable organizations to AA for cirrhosis patients, a societal shortcoming that calls for creativity on your part.

Where can you find other cirrhosis patients that would be interested in sharing their experiences with you? You can start with your doctor. Ask if any of her patients would be interested in forming an organization similar to AA. Ask for the names and telephone numbers of any patients who would be interested. Religious organizations are another possibility. Talk to your minister, priest, or rabbi. Ask them to make an appeal to their congregation. If all else fails, you can always run a newspaper ad, but doing so requires caution, since it could set you up for abuse at the hands of unscrupulous persons who may seek to exploit your condition for financial gain.

One of the newest additions to the support network are online Web sites that allow patients to discuss their particular problems and concerns in a public forum that encourages debate through e-mail exchanges. These sites are easy to find. Simply google "cirrhosis support group" and visit the various sites until you find one that appeals to you.

I visited a liver failure support group at http://forums.delphiforums.com and I was impressed with the exchanges that I read. A forty-nine-year-old grandmother named Donna expressed her frustration at feeling so isolated, despite the fact that she has a husband, a daughter, three grandchildren, two sisters, and a mother. It frustrates her that one of her sisters insists that she could cure herself if only she prayed harder, and the other sister thinks she is a "downer" because she is often depressed. She reached out on the Internet in the hope that other cirrhosis patients would understand her frustrations.

Sites such as this can be a wonderful tool for reaching out to others with cirrhosis. However, it is prudent to use the same level of caution on the Internet that you would use speaking to a stranger on a street corner. Never give out personal information to strangers that would allow them to "steal" your identity. By that, I mean keep your Social Security number, your birth date, and your middle and mother's maiden name private. There is no legitimate reason for anyone in an Internet support group to ask you for such information.

Tips for getting the support you need

It may seem unfair that your cirrhosis has imposed itself on your family life in such an unwanted way, but there is nothing fair about the disease, and the less time you spend contemplating that, the better off you will be.

Here are some survival tips I hope will be helpful:

- ○ Don't try to reinvent your relationships with your partner, children, or parents to accommodate your new perspective on life. Accept them for who they are and don't try to change them. Allow them to provide you with the kind of support they have always offered you.
- ○ Seek out other cirrhosis patients to satisfy your need for conversation about your disease. Schedule regular meetings with them, just as you would with a social organization. Do this and you will not feel quite so alone in the world.
- ○ Get involved in public education about the disease. Volunteer to speak to students about the dangers of alcohol and drug use, improperly handled food, etc.
- ○ Volunteer at your local hospital to assist with children who have cirrhosis. It may help you feel more positive about your condition.

IN A SENTENCE:

> *Reach out to others for support.*

learning

Insurance and Financial Planning

IF YOU thought hearing the news that you have cirrhosis was a shock that left you weak in the knees, unfortunately, that is nothing compared to the shock you will encounter when you start calculating how you will pay for the medical treatment you will need to survive your illness. For starters, if you do not already have health insurance, it is unlikely that an insurance company will issue you a policy after diagnosis. Even if you do have health insurance, the costs can still add up, depending on what procedures and medications your policy will cover.

Within weeks of my diagnosis, my insurance company dramatically increased my monthly premiums. Included with the notice was a statement that the insurance company reserved the right to further increase my premiums as it sees fit. (The notice made me realize how foolish it is to allow private enterprise to operate our national health-care system. No other industrialized nation allows such a system to exist.)

If uninsured, to pay for your treatment, you will need to use your savings, mortgage your home, rely on credit, or borrow money from friends and relatives. Unless you live below the poverty level, or have filed for bankruptcy, there will be no government safety net to help you with your expenses. Although hospitals are required to perform emergency services to indigent patients, your cirrhosis will not qualify you for treatment unless you are experiencing serious complications, such as bleeding.

Despite the apparent roadblocks, it is essential that you explore all your options. Giving up because of financial difficulties is not an option if you want to overcome your disease. The best option is to press ahead. If you don't have health insurance, you're not alone. U.S. Census data puts the number of uninsured Americans at between forty and forty-five million. Some are parents whose employers do not provide health insurance. Some are self-employed parents who cannot afford to pay for an individual policy. Almost six million of them are mothers of children under nineteen who earn too much to qualify for poverty assistance and not enough to afford health insurance.

One study found that about one-third of people without health insurance had annual incomes of $25,000 to $50,000. These are hardworking people, for the most part, whose families would be thrown into chaos by a major medical expense. They live day to day, paycheck to paycheck. Not surprisingly, the percentage of Americans without health insurance varies considerably from state to state. In Texas, nearly 25 percent of residents are without health insurance, according to U.S. Census data. Other high-percentage states are New Mexico (21 percent), Oklahoma (18 percent), Louisiana (19 percent), and California (20 percent). The states with percentages below 10 percent—Wisconsin, Vermont, North Dakota, South Dakota, Rhode Island, Delaware, Iowa, and Minnesota—still have work to do, since their numbers are all close to 10 percent.

Even if you have insurance, you could still run into problems, depending on whether you have an individual policy or whether it is part of a group policy offered by your employer. Your insurance company cannot drop you because you have a chronic illness, but it can raise your rates on a regular basis to the point where you can no longer afford to pay the premiums.

A minority of Americans (about 15 percent) have disability insurance — and if that is your situation, congratulations on your good fortune—but once a person has been diagnosed with cirrhosis, it is too late to sign up for that type of policy.

Cirrhosis patients have two major adversaries—the disease itself and a health-care system that requires a considerable financial investment for recovery. If you believe that life is worth fighting for—and I sincerely hope that is the case—then your only true option is to press forward in both areas. Don't give up. You *can* do this!

Tips to help you find peace of mind

So what's the best way to financially prepare for your health care? Once you have been diagnosed with cirrhosis, you have two choices: you can withdraw into yourself and obsess over your bad luck—or you can take charge of those things that are still under your control and plan for the future. Obviously, it is the latter choice that will offer you the most health benefits. Taking action is the key to both physical and emotional good health—and that goes for your finances, too.

Whether you have health insurance or not, you'll first need to organize your finances to determine your health-care budget. In the beginning, it will be difficult for you to anticipate your upcoming monthly medical expenses. It will depend on how often your doctor wants to see you, how often she wants to run tests, and whether medications will be prescribed. What you can do is figure out how much per month you can spend on health-care costs without dipping into your savings. Once you have done that, you should take stock of your assets, including your savings account, and calculate how much of your net worth can be converted to cash on relatively short notice.

How much money will you need? The answer to that depends on whether you have insurance or not. If you don't have insurance, you should figure on spending about $15,000 the first year and $5,000 to $8,000 a year after that for doctor's visits, tests, and medication, assuming you have no major complications that will require surgery. If the worst happens—and your cirrhosis progresses to complete liver failure—you will need a liver transplant, the cost of which can vary from $150,000 to $250,000. If the surgery is successful, you probably will have to take antirejection medication for the rest of your life and the cost could run to several thousand dollars a month, depending on the medication prescribed.

If you do have insurance, you will need to meet with your employer's insurance representative, or, in the case of private insurance, with a company representative, to go over your policy's inclusions and exclusions. You should ask questions about the following:

- What is your policy's lifetime value? It is probably more than enough to pay your bills, but it's best to receive confirmation of that.
- What are your options in choosing your own physicians? If your policy is implemented by an HMO, your freedom of choice in selecting physicians and treatment centers may be severely limited. Ask for a clear directive on what choices you are permitted under your policy.
- Is there a limitation on the number of tests your physician can order each year? If there is a limit, you need to advise your physician so that she can better plan your treatment.
- Does your policy cover the costs of a liver transplant? Most insurance companies will pay the cost of a liver transplant, but you should ask for confirmation of that so that you do not encounter any last-minute surprises.
- Does your policy cover the costs of postsurgery antirejection medications? Many policies do not cover those expenses, so you should find that out now so that you can plan for that potential expense.
- Is your policy convertible to a private policy? You need to have that information now so that you can be prepared if your employment terminates.

If you have problems with your insurance company paying for certain drugs or tests, you should discuss it with your physician. She may be able to convince the insurance company to pay the costs, or, failing that, she may be able to enroll you in free clinical trials conducted by pharmaceutical companies. The trials are held to test new medications before they are put on the market, and enrollment in the trials often means free tests in addition to free medication. Before you agree to be part of a clinical trial, you should ask the following questions:

- What are the side effects of the medication?
- If, after enrolling in the program, you decide it is not right for you, will you be able to drop out of the trial without obligation?
- Will your trial involve the use of placebos? If so—and you end up on the placebo list—will you be able to receive the drug being tested after the trial is concluded? If the answer is no, you must come to terms with the possibility that you might undergo a months-long

trial without ever receiving actual medication. Talk to your physician about how that would affect the progress of your disease.

○ Some pharmaceutical companies offer their medications free of charge to needy patients who require the drugs for survival. Talk to your physician about that possibility. She may be willing to approach the pharmaceutical company on your behalf.

Government entitlement programs

Your year of birth will determine when you are eligible to qualify for Social Security benefits at full retirement age, but regardless of your age you must have earned forty credits to be able to qualify for benefits.

Provided you have the credits, your full retirement age was sixty-four if you were born in 1937 or earlier. The retirement age inches upward in two-month increments for those born between 1938 and 1942, and changes to age sixty-six for those born between 1943 and 1954. If you were born between 1955 and 1959, the retirement age increases at two-month intervals until it reaches age sixty-seven for those born in 1960 or later.

If you have earned forty credits, you are entitled to receive early retirement benefits at age sixty-two, but your benefits will be permanently reduced based on the number of months during which you receive benefits before you reach full retirement age.

Of course, the most important entitlement benefit you can receive is Medicare, which will begin when you reach full retirement age. It is recommended that you apply for Medicare at least three months prior to your full retirement-age birthday.

Medicaid is a federal-state program that is designed to provide health care for people with low incomes. Requirements vary from state to state and in some locations it is limited solely to children or single-parent families with children. To find out if you are eligible, you should contact your local social services department.

If you are a veteran, you may qualify for medical benefits and disability payments. Liver transplants are routinely approved by the Veterans Administration, so if you are a veteran you should contact the Veterans Administration Regional Office and talk to them about their transplant program, even if you have not previously applied for veteran's benefits.

In addition to the retirement benefits administered by the Social Security Administration, there are two disability programs for which you may qualify—Social Security Disability Insurance (SSDI) and Supplemental Security Income (SSI).

Both programs recognize cirrhosis as a disability, but for you to receive benefits under either program you will have to experience serious complications. Massive hemorrhage due to **esophageal varices** would qualify you for benefits, but they would be limited to three years, after which you would have to be reevaluated; if your varices are no longer a problem, your disability benefits will be terminated.

Other complications that will, at least, give you a basis to make an application for benefits include ascites that are not attributable to other causes, encephalopathy caused by cirrhosis, or bilirubin levels of 2.5 mg that persist for three months or more. An added requirement of the SSI program is that the patient be "indigent," defined as having little or no income and assets of less than $2,000.

According to the Social Security Administration, only 37 percent of patients who apply for disability payments are approved. That number jumps to 55 percent after appeals are taken into consideration. These figures alone are a good argument for hiring a lawyer to represent you in your application.

If you feel that you might qualify for Social Security disability benefits, you should contact the Social Security office and request information about how to apply.

Long-term care

As a cirrhosis patient, you may feel fine at the moment, but the nature of the disease is that it sometimes follows a progression of complications, beginning with ascites and bleeding varices—and ending with kidney and liver failure and coma. None of those complications may ever happen to you. You may live to age ninety and die of a stroke while doing twenty laps in the swimming pool. But the one thing you don't want is to play the odds, which is why the time to plan for your long-term health care is now.

Is your insurance adequate to provide for your financial needs? If not, you should consider putting your assets into a trust under the administration of someone you trust. That way, if you become incapacitated and unable to handle your own finances, there will be someone in place with the authority to make decisions in your best interests.

If you do not have enough assets to make a trust worthwhile, yet you own your own home, talk to a lawyer about how you can protect your home in the event you become incapacitated. In addition, you should also become familiar with your rights regarding federal and state assistance programs. If you develop complications such as ascites or bleeding varices, you may become eligible for federal disability benefits.

Make a list of what you anticipate your needs will be over the next few years and put thought into how you can fill those needs.

For example, you may be able to go to work and carry on with your profession for many years, so it will be your time at home alone that is more important to factor into your needs. Every cirrhosis patient should make arrangements for someone to live at home with them, whether it is a relative, a romantic partner, or a friend.

If you can afford it, another option would be to hire home health-care workers. As your disease progresses, you will need another set of hands, eyes, and ears. Aside from needing someone around in case of emergencies, you may need someone to drive you to appointments or travel with you to a transplant center. Again, many cirrhosis patients live long, full lives without ever needing anything resembling nursing care at home, but it's best to be prepared, just in case.

Also, at some point, you will want to examine your options for advance directives, including instructions for a living will or any other matter you want handled in the event that you are incapacitated.

Advance directives

> I have this fear that I will be in a coma
> and none of my family members
> will have the courage to pull the plug.
>
> —JEFFREY K.

Advance directives are road maps for how you want your affairs handled. It may take the form of a living will or a durable power of attorney or a "do not resuscitate" order, all as defined by you. These are means for you to appoint someone to direct your care in the event you are incapacitated and unable to do so.

A living will is crucial for every cirrhosis patient. Even though it's likely your eventual death will be the result of another, unrelated condition, in the event that something does go awry, there is a small chance you could suffer liver or kidney failure of a type that leaves you in a coma.

If that were the case, what would you want to happen at that point? Would you want to be kept alive for as long as medically possible? Or would you prefer that you be taken off life support once your doctor says recovery is unlikely?

If you are in a relationship, the responsibility for making that decision naturally falls on the spouse. However, if you have no spouse, you will need to decide who will take that responsibility. Your sister or brother? Your daughter? Your ex-wife or ex-husband? Your best friend? This is not necessarily an easy matter. The most realistic choices are the doctor who is treating you (she has spent a great deal of time and effort keeping you alive and will not give up without good reason), the lawyer who drew up your will (if it is someone you have had a long-term relationship with), or a relative who you feel could handle the pressure of this decision. Difficult to think about? Yes, but absolutely necessary.

You probably never realized that having a serious illness required so much work. As unpleasant as it may be to deal with insurance problems, disability applications, and advance directives, it is a part of your life now and it is to your advantage to throw yourself into that work with the same intensity you muster for the treatment of your disease. View it as a challenge, not a curse, and you will find a way to prevail.

IN A SENTENCE:

> *Financial planning can give you peace of mind.*

FIRST-MONTH MILESTONE

What You Should Have Done by Now

- ○ YOU HAVE LEARNED HOW YOUR LIVER WORKS.

- ○ YOU HAVE SELECTED THE DOCTOR(S) WHO WILL SEE YOU THROUGH YOUR TREATMENT.

- ○ YOU HAVE TOLD LOVED ONES ABOUT YOUR ILLNESS.

- ○ YOU HAVE UNDERGONE A VARIETY OF TESTS, INCLUDING A SONOGRAM, CT SCAN, BLOOD TESTS, AND BIOPSY.

- ○ YOU KNOW YOUR CHILD-PUGH SCORE.

- ○ YOU HAVE EVALUATED YOUR FINANCIAL SITUATION.

- ○ YOU HAVE TAKEN SOME TIME OFF TO DEAL WITH YOUR FEELINGS ABOUT YOUR DIAGNOSIS.

Finding a Therapist

> *Getting cirrhosis is a little bit like*
> *being a Democrat your entire life,*
> *only to wake up one day*
> *to find that you are a Republican.*
>
> —TONY P.

IF YOU'RE having difficulty coping with the changes in your life, or simply want to share the feelings you're having, you might wish to find a therapist to talk to during the first year of your illness, especially if you are feeling alone or isolated because of your condition. If so, seek a licensed therapist who has experience counseling individuals who have been diagnosed with serious illnesses. You will be surprised how beneficial having a therapist can be in the treatment of your disease.

Katie G. cried in her doctor's office when she was told that she had cirrhosis. A registered nurse, she understood the seriousness of the diagnosis. Her disease was caused by hepatitis C, which she and her doctor guessed probably originated from a needle that pricked her skin after she withdrew blood from an infected patient.

After two weeks of sleepless nights and frequent outbursts of crying, she finally took a friend's advice and went to see a licensed social worker who specialized in treating health-related anxiety. Her main problem was that her job exposed her to ill individuals on a daily basis. She understood what could go wrong in people with cirrhosis because she had witnessed it firsthand.

The social worker was able to help her by pointing out that she was burdened by an excessive amount of negative information. As part of the therapy, Katie was encouraged to focus on the many victories she had witnessed as a nurse. Many cirrhosis patients live long, happy lives and end up dying of heart attacks or strokes. Katie understood that intellectually, but it was only through therapy that she was able to accept it emotionally. Eventually, she was able to come to terms with her illness. Although she continued to complain to her doctor about her bad luck, the crying stopped and those who knew her best marveled at her new attitude.

If therapy is appropriate for you, there are several different types of therapists for you to choose from: psychologists, psychiatrists, or social workers. Psychologists have doctorates or master's degrees and they tend to focus more on those aspects of your life that relate to your behavior in certain situations, such as being obsessive or compulsive about your illness. Psychiatrists are medical doctors who specialize in more serious problems that sometimes require prescription medication. Social workers have doctorates or master's degrees and they focus on the significant relationships in your life, whether they fall within the categories of family, romantic attachments, or employment.

Before you engage the services of a therapist, you should confer with the physician who is treating your cirrhosis and ask for his or her suggestions. If you are showing no symptoms of mental problems due to the toxic effects of your cirrhosis—hallucinations, memory lapses, etc.—your physician will probably recommend that you see a psychologist or a social worker. That choice can be further narrowed by an understanding of whether you are exhibiting obsessive or compulsive behavior or whether you are having problems controlling your emotions, in which case a psychologist would probably be the best choice for you. If what you need is someone to counsel you about your own acceptance of the disease or your relationships with friends and family members, then a social worker would be more appropriate.

One word of advice: whomever you choose as your therapist, do so after meeting with more than one candidate—and steer clear of therapists who are known to you socially or are members of your religious institution. Your therapist should be a total stranger who has no information about you other than what is derived from his interviews with you. When you meet with various therapists to decide who will be the best fit for you, view those encounters as you would any other relationship in your life. Choose the person with whom you feel the strongest connection.

If, during your first interview, the therapist seems distracted or takes personal calls, or asks, after being told that you have cirrhosis, why you feel a need to see a therapist, then you know you have not formed a therapy connection. If, on the other hand, the therapist makes strong eye contact with you and asks you questions that indicate that he understands why you are seeking help, those are signs of a connection.

What should I discuss with a therapist?

You may have reservations about sharing your innermost thoughts with others, especially strangers; but since the object of therapy is to free you from the negative baggage attached to those innermost thoughts, you must enter the process with an open mind and a willingness to discuss the issues that are causing you pain.

Among the things you might discuss with a therapist are:

○ How you think your illness has affected your relationships with others. For example, do you sense that your significant other is withdrawing from you because of your illness? Is your family providing you with too much comfort, or not enough?

○ How you think your illness has affected your employment. Are you concerned that your employer will feel that you can no longer do the work required of your position? Are you concerned that you may be fired because of your health-care expenses?

○ How you think your illness has affected your view of life in general. Are you reluctant to commit to projects that will require your long-term involvement?

○ How you think the stress associated with your illness is affecting your decision-making. Are you making bad decisions about loved ones, finances, etc.? Are you making mistakes that you would not have made before you became ill?

○ How you think your illness has made you feel alone in the universe. Don't be afraid to tell your therapist, "I have never felt so alone in my life." Loneliness is difficult to discuss with loved ones since they will invariably interpret your feelings as a failing on their part. That won't be a problem with your therapist, who will understand the source of your feelings.

How long will therapy take?

It will take as long as it takes, and not a minute sooner. Therapy is not a product that you can pick up at a drive-through window. The odds are that you had problems, however minor, that could have benefited from therapy even before you were diagnosed with cirrhosis.

Therapy is the means through which you will come to terms with your past—and accept your future. There is no quick cure for that. It could take months, perhaps years, to reach a plateau of comfortable resolution. The important thing to understand is that the better you feel about yourself during your treatment, the better your odds for a successful outcome. A positive attitude is one of the most powerful drugs at your disposal.

IN A SENTENCE:

> Talking with a therapist about your condition can improve your emotional and physical health.

learning

What Are My Treatment Options?

> *The biggest surprise I've had as a cirrhosis*
> *patient has been the long-term approach*
> *my doctor has taken in my treatment.*
> *He told me all along that there was no*
> *quick fix, but it took me a year to believe him.*
>
> —SHILOH W.

YOUR SPECIFIC treatment options largely depend on the cause of your cirrhosis. From the moment that you were first diagnosed with cirrhosis, your options were all in place, waiting for your disease to reveal its true colors. Your doctor probably did not discuss treatment options with you in those early days because the available options are all cause-specific—and until such time as the cause is understood, there is little your doctor can do in the way of treatment.

Whatever the cause, cirrhosis is a disease that requires a lot of patience to treat. It takes the liver a relatively long time to heal. Victories usually come in small increments. Once your doctor sees evidence of healing, you may find it surprising that instead of asking you to come into the office once a month, as you have done from the beginning, he or she may not schedule you for another office visit for three to six months. In other words, the better your liver functions, the less your doctor will want to see you.

"There is no single 'magic bullet' to treat cirrhosis," writes Dr. Sanjiv Chopra in his book *Dr. Sanjiv Chopra's Liver Book*. "The best we can do is to limit any further damage by managing the underlying disease that caused the cirrhosis in the first place. The different therapies that are available thus vary widely depending on what caused the cirrhosis and on which (if any) complications have developed."

Alcohol-related cirrhosis

Of course, as you've learned by now, the successful treatment of cirrhosis caused by alcohol abuse depends on the patient's willingness to stop drinking. If the patient is unable (for reasons of dependency) or unwilling to abstain from alcohol use, there is little that can be done to improve the patient's prognosis. However, if the patient is able and willing to abstain from alcohol use, the odds are excellent that the cirrhosis will not progress beyond its current level of scarring. In that case, vitamins may be the only recommended treatment, unless complications to the initial scarring present themselves.

In some instances, supportive medical care may be necessary for individuals who suffer withdrawal complications after terminating their alcohol use, but the medical care will be directed toward the withdrawal symptoms and not the cirrhosis. Once the patient has been stabilized, in-patient rehabilitation may be required for at least one month, along with psychotherapy and involvement in Alcoholics Anonymous.

The most difficult thing for patients with alcohol-related cirrhosis to accept is that the treatment of their disease is entirely dependent on their ability to stop drinking. In other words, there comes a point when it is the patient's addiction—and not the cirrhosis—that must be considered the most threatening disease.

Viral hepatitis—hepatitis B, C, and D

If your cirrhosis was caused by viral hepatitis, your treatment will focus on drug therapy that targets the virus. If you have hepatitis B, you probably will be given one of four drugs—interferon, adefovir, entecavir, or lamivudine. Interferon is produced in the human body in small amounts to fight viral and bacterial infections. Since it cannot be produced in the body in large enough quantities to take on a disease like hepatitis B, doctors prescribe the interferon in dosages strong enough to give the immune system a boost. It is sold under three trade names—Infergen, Intron A, and Roferon A. There are two forms of interferon—Peg-Intron and Pegasys. The doses and treatment durations vary based on the type of interferon.

Lamivudine was used for many years to treat AIDS before it was approved as a treatment for hepatitis B. Unlike interferon, which has troublesome side effects such as lowering the patient's resistance to infection or increasing the patient's susceptibility to eye problems, lamivudine has no serious side effects. Its main drawback is that in up to one-fourth of the people who take it for one year, the hepatitis B virus becomes drug resistant—and the long-term effect of that is currently unknown.

Interferon is also a possibility if you have hepatitis C, along with a drug named ribavirin. Typically the two drugs are combined into one medication that is sold under the name Rebetron. The success rate with Rebetron is high—an encouraging 70 percent under certain conditions—but doctors differ in their opinion of when to begin the treatment. If the disease is mild, some doctors prefer to adopt a wait-and-see attitude regarding treatment. Others start treatment right away.

"I endorse this option [Rebetron treatment] for most patients if they have a lot of stability in their lives; that is, if they're not overstressed by a demanding job, under pressure to finish a PhD dissertation, or waking up every few hours at night to feed a newborn, and if they're not drinking alcohol and don't have any trouble keeping medical appointments," says Dr. Sanjiv Chopra. "If you take interferon and ribavirin therapy, but experience significant side effects and inconveniences, you can talk with your doctor about stopping treatment and take comfort in the knowledge that eventually better medicines will become available."

If you have hepatitis D, your doctor may prescribe interferon, but the drug's effectiveness with this strain of hepatitis is not nearly as encouraging as it is with hepatitis B and C patients. For the most part, treatment is supportive in that it will be directed toward whatever complications develop. You will either get well on your own or your disease will progress to the point where you will need a liver transplant.

The important thing to remember about hepatitis treatment is that if you are fortunate enough to stop the virus and the inflammation caused by the virus, you will still have to deal with the by-product of the virus, namely cirrhosis. The good news is that once you stop the virus, you stop the progress of your cirrhosis. On rare occasions, interferon has even been known to make it possible for scar tissue to regenerate into healthy tissue, but you cannot count on that happening in your case.

If you are not currently experiencing complications from cirrhosis, there is a good chance you never will, provided you do not abuse your new lease on life. It is essential that you never drink alcohol or use IV drugs. If you have not been vaccinated for hepatitis A, you should arrange to do so immediately. Meanwhile, you should be careful not to eat restaurant foods that are handled without utensils by food workers (salad, for example). And you should make certain that your doctor screens any prescription drugs you might take for unrelated illnesses for potential side effects.

Generally speaking, if you knock down the hepatitis virus, the prognosis for your cirrhosis is good—and you are likely to enjoy a normal life span.

Autoimmune hepatitis

Treatment usually begins immediately after a biopsy confirms a diagnosis of autoimmune hepatitis. Time is a factor since the disease, if untreated, can escalate rapidly to liver failure for which the *only* option may be a liver transplant. However, patients with autoimmune hepatitis presenting in an acute stage can be easily treated with prednisone, a steroid, and Imuran (azathioprine), a drug used to fight organ rejection in kidney transplants. Prednisone is the major player, with Imuran used primarily to enhance the effect of the prednisone.

The initial dose of prednisone may be anywhere from 10 to 50 mg and the initial dose of Imuran will usually be in the 50 to 100 mg range. Those amounts are usually tapered over the next six to twenty-four months, depending on the patient's reaction to the drugs.

The majority of patients on this drug therapy (some experts put it at 70 to 80 percent) experience normal ALT and AST enzyme levels after several months of treatment, an indication that their liver inflammation has gone into a type of remission. The real test comes after the medications are stopped. Some patients remain in remission and can stay off their medication for months or even years. Others need a low-maintenance dose of 2 to 5 mg of prednisone a day for an indefinite period of time. In general, the patient's chances of survival are very good over the long term.

My experience with the prednisone/Imuran combo has been very encouraging. I started off with 40 mg of prednisone, which was quickly reduced to 30 mg and then dropped to 10 mg per day. My blood tests came back normal in all categories.

Side effects of prednisone include mood changes, increased appetite, indigestion, difficulty sleeping, swelling in the feet or legs, vomit that looks like coffee grounds, headache, glaucoma or cataracts, acne, diabetes, prolonged sore throat or colds, and fever. Side effects of azathioprine include stomach upset, diarrhea, vomiting, rash, muscle aches, and bleeding or bruising. The risk of side effects is linked to dosage and the length of time the patient is on the medication. Patients with cirrhosis are more likely to experience side effects than patients who have not yet experienced liver damage.

Nonalcoholic fatty liver disease (NAFLD)

Most of the people who have NAFLD are asymptomatic—or if they do have symptoms, they are typically vague enough to be referred to simply as fatigue and weakness. However, there is one characteristic that occurs more than any other—obesity.

Not all obese people have NAFLD, and not everyone who has NAFLD is obese (a sedentary lifestyle and a diet rich in fat and sugar can lead to fatty liver, even in people of normal weight), but the weight factor is prevalent enough in patients with this form of cirrhosis that it will be the doctor's first concern. Sometimes medications are prescribed for weight loss. Some of the most frequently prescribed weight-loss medications are Adipex-P (phentermine), Meridia (sibutramine) and Xenical (orlistat).

There is no standard medical treatment for NAFLD, but the most common approach to controlling the disease involves the use of ursodiol (Actigall), a drug commonly used to treat gallstones, and the use of vitamins E and C, since they are believed to reduce liver damage caused by oxidants.

For more on NAFLD, please see Obesity and Cirrhosis, page TK.

Vitamin A–related cirrhosis

The liver stores more than 90 percent of your body's Vitamin A supply. That is normally a good thing, but problems can arise if you either exceed the recommended daily allowance of the vitamin or consume alcohol on a regular basis.

The recommended daily allowance of vitamin A is 700 RAE (retinol activity equivalent) per day for women and 900 RAE per day for men. The foods that contain the highest amounts of vitamin A are sweet potatoes (1,400 RAE per half cup), carrots (1,015 RAE per medium-sized carrot), turnip greens (100 RAE per half cup), and fat-free milk (150 RAE per cup). Most multivitamins contain 700 to 900 RAE of vitamin A in each tablet.

For some reason, alcohol intensifies the toxic effect of vitamin A, so if you are in the habit of taking a multivitamin and like to drink beer with your sweet potatoes (1 cup), carrots (3 cups) and cantaloupe (1 cup), you are looking at an intake of nearly 7,000 RAE of vitamin A, seven to eight times the recommended allowance—and enough to jump-start cirrhosis in your unsuspecting liver. Also capable of causing cirrhosis are megadoses of vitamin A, of the type you sometimes see advocated by health enthusiasts.

There is no specific treatment for cirrhosis caused by vitamin A. However, if you abstain from drinking alcohol, stop taking vitamin supplements containing vitamin A, and curtail your intake of vitamin A–rich foods until natural levels of the vitamin resume inside the liver, your cirrhosis hopefully will not progress beyond its current level.

Prescription or nonprescription drug-related liver disease

Tylenol (acetaminophen) is one of the biggest contributors to drug-related acute hepatitis and fulminant liver failure, especially when mixed with alcohol. It is for that reason that Tylenol has become a popular means of attempting suicide.

Ironically, doctors are not hesitant to prescribe recommended doses of Tylenol to nondrinking patients with existing cirrhosis since it is felt that the drug is a more acceptable alternative to aspirin, which can cause gastrointestinal bleeding.

There are literally hundreds of prescription drugs that can cause acute hepatitis, liver failure, or cirrhosis, including Valium, Motrin, tetracycline,

Dilantin, Avandia, and Tamoxifen—and dozens of over-the-counter or illegal drugs such as aspirin and cocaine—and the only treatment option that you have is to stop taking the drugs.

Whether you survive a drug-related liver failure or cirrhosis will depend on your liver's ability to purge the drugs from your system, and it will depend on the amount of damage caused by the drugs. Obviously, your prognosis is better if your liver can eliminate the drugs before cirrhosis becomes evident.

There are basically two scenarios for patients who have developed cirrhosis as a result of a drug reaction: they either enter an acute phase that leads to liver failure and a complete shutdown of the organ, necessitating a transplant, or their liver eliminates the drug from their system and leaves them with a chronic form of cirrhosis that is unlikely to worsen unless complications unexpectedly develop.

Wilson's disease

Wilson's disease is a genetic disorder that develops from copper poisoning. Small amounts of copper are essential to the body; it is used as needed and excreted. However, some individuals are unable to excrete the copper absorbed by their body and it accumulates until it reaches toxic levels. The body's inability to process copper usually begins at birth, but does not display symptoms until adolescence, when the first sign of trouble is usually jaundice, vomiting of blood, and abdominal pain. Some patients have trouble walking, talking, or swallowing, and they may show signs of mental illness such as homicidal or suicidal behavior.

This condition is often misdiagnosed as infectious hepatitis or infectious mononucleosis. This is a treatable disease, but only if it is diagnosed in a timely manner. Any delay in treatment can result in irreversible liver damage. Treatment consists of removing excess copper from the system and preventing its reaccumulation. Drugs used to treat Wilson's disease include Galzin (zinc acetate), Cuprimine (penicillamine), Depen and Syprine (trientine). There is more about this disease in the chapter about children (Month 6).

Primary biliary cirrhosis

Primary biliary cirrhosis (PBC) is an autoimmune disorder similar to autoimmune hepatitis that is characterized by the destruction of the bile ducts within the liver. Why it attacks the cells in the bile ducts and not the liver cells is a mystery. One consequence of the attack is that the bile acids run out of the damaged bile ducts and inflame the surrounding liver tissue, thus causing cirrhosis.

No one knows exactly what causes PBC, but it is thought to occur in people with a genetic susceptibility to the disease. Caucasians, especially those from northern Europe, are the most likely to come down with the disease. Africans and Indians rarely get the disease. Women are far more at risk than men, with women accounting for about 95 percent of cases. While it most commonly attacks people aged forty to sixty, it has been diagnosed in people in their twenties and in their nineties. Researchers feel the most likely "triggers" for the disease are environmental factors such as cigarette smoke, tainted water, viral and bacterial infections, and prescription drugs.

Treatment of PBC is aimed at slowing the progression of cirrhosis and controlling the symptoms associated with the disease. Drugs sometimes used to treat PBC include prednisone, cyclosporine (an antirejection drug), and chlorambucil, a drug often used in chemotherapy. In her practice, Dr. Melissa Palmer has found that three drugs have proved the most effective— Actigall or Urso (ursodiol), which has been approved by the FDA for the treatment of PBC; methotrexate; and colchicine, an anti-inflammatory drug that has been reported to reduce scarring in the liver, but not necessarily to reduce inflammation. Dr. Howard Worman considers Actigall or Urso to be a safe drug with few side effects. He does not consider it a cure, but he feels that it has proven effective in slowing the progression of the disease. The recommended dose is 13 to 15 mg per kilogram of body weight. Dr. Sanjiv Chopra treats most of his PBC patients with Actigall, which he finds often relieves the itching associated with the disease. His preferred dosage is 900 to 1,200 mg a day. He reports that Actigall can reduce the risk of complications such as esophageal varices. Dr. Fredric Regenstein considers Urso a harmless drug that may slow the progression of PBC, along with low doses of colchicine (another safe drug of questionable benefit), but he feels that the other drugs mentioned have side effects that may outweigh any potential benefit offered for the treatment of PBC.

While there is no cure for PBC, other than a liver transplant, it progresses over a period of many years and patients who have it often die of unrelated diseases.

Hemochromatosis

Hemochromatosis is an inherited disease that primarily affects individuals of European descent. It is caused by an abnormal accumulation of iron in the liver and other organs. Since the disease is very slow to develop, usually over a period of many years, it is usually not diagnosed until complications arise. Symptoms include arthritis, especially in the hands, chronic fatigue, abnormal menstruation, and a reduction in the sex drive.

If the disease is diagnosed early, there is an effective treatment called phlebotomy, which is probably better known by the ancient term *bloodletting*. The idea is to draw off enough blood to lower the red blood cell count to a level that is slightly below normal. It sounds archaic, but it works.

If the disease is not diagnosed until cirrhosis has already occurred, phlebotomy performed on a periodic basis may prevent serious complications from developing, but it cannot reverse the cirrhosis.

Herbal-related cirrhosis

I discuss the possible benefits of herbs on pages 197–199, but this space is devoted to herbs that are known to cause liver damage. Obviously, no one ever sets out to get cirrhosis of the liver from an herb. What usually happens is that a person uses an herb to treat a seemingly mild condition such as joint pain or a stomachache—and ends up with a life-threatening liver disease. Whether that occurs after one use or several uses depends on the herb and its potency.

Comfrey, sometimes used as a natural means to treat stomach ulcers, is an example. Available as a tea or in tablet or capsule form, its alkaloid compounds have been linked to cirrhosis of the liver. Other herbs that have been associated with liver disease include buckthorn, black cohosh, sassafras, sweet clover, kava, green tea leaf, germander, sarsaparilla, ragwort, nutmeg, and pokeweed.

Any treatment for herb-related cirrhosis begins with the removal of the herb from the patient's diet and proceeds to traditional remedies for any complications that arise. The progress of the cirrhosis may be stopped, but the scar tissue itself will remain for life.

Cryptogenic cirrhosis

Cryptogenic cirrhosis is the name doctors give to cirrhosis for which there is no apparent cause. Since there is no known virus, toxin, or organ malfunction that can be directly linked to cryptogenic cirrhosis, its origins remain a mystery (hence, as mentioned above, the name "crypto"). The treatment consists of avoiding substances such as alcohol, prescription and nonprescription drugs, certain herbs and vitamins, risky food sources, and other risk factors that might cause further damage.

IN A SENTENCE:

The treatment for cirrhosis is based on its cause.

How Much Should I Exercise?

> *Before I was diagnosed with cirrhosis*
> *I used to run every morning. Now I don't*
> *know what to do. I'm tired most of the time*
> *and I don't feel like running. Yet I feel like I*
> *should be doing some sort of exercise.*
>
> —BETH C.

REGULAR EXERCISE is one of the two most important things you can do to assist your doctor with your treatment, the second being maintaining a healthy diet. Patients who exercise on a regular basis not only feel better, but they often respond better to treatment than those who do not.

There is also the matter of weight gain. Many of the drugs used to treat cirrhosis and the diseases that cause cirrhosis have weight gain as a side effect. If you have ever known a liver patient who is on a drug such as prednisone, you are familiar with the fatty, "moon" face that the drug can sometimes produce as a result of weight gain. You may already be at that point yourself. That has not happened to me—at least not yet—and I am certain that a major reason is the fact that I have exercised on a daily basis for the past thirty years and I did not allow my diagnosis slow me down.

Be sure to talk with your doctor before you embark on any exercise regime, especially if you have been sedentary for the past few years.

The benefits of walking

I think walking is the perfect exercise for cirrhosis patients, not just because it is the safest—not a small issue for people who may be over-weight and thus already taxing their heart and organs—but because it is the most effective way to maintain weight control once the desired number of pounds has been lost.

Not only does walking allow you to burn several hundred calories a day, it boosts your metabolic rate for the remainder of the day, a secondary ben-efit that results in the burning of even more calories.

I walk thirty minutes each day. The experts recommend that amount to prevent adding new pounds, and sixty minutes each day to burn fat. Jogging and running, while fine for lean people with healthy cardiovascular systems, is counterproductive for overweight individuals; it makes injuries more likely and it impedes the body's ability to transfer energy from fat cells.

A study conducted by health psychologists—and published in the *American Journal of Health Promotion*—found that people who live in the sub-urbs weigh more than those who live in cities. People living in a sprawling, suburban county in Ohio were found to weigh, on average, six pounds more—and walked seventy-nine minutes less each month—than people who lived in New York County (Manhattan). The researchers attributed that difference to the fact that the people in Manhattan walked and rode their bikes more than the people who lived in the suburbs.

Walking will allow you to control your weight and reduce your total body fat. Your total body fat was probably not much of an issue for you before you were diagnosed with cirrhosis, but it certainly should be now. That is because excess body fat makes it more difficult for your liver to do its work. When you reduce your body fat, you also reduce the fat content of your liver—and, if your liver enzymes are elevated, that can result in a reduction in your AST and ALT scores.

Walking will give you an energy boost. Since fatigue is one of the most common symptoms of cirrhosis, or liver disease in general, energy is a prized commodity. If you feel tired all the time, or if you have problems getting the sleep you need, walking will help. The suggestion that you should exercise to combat your fatigue may sound ridiculous, but it works. Sure, you may be tired when you return from your walk, but that tiredness will be of short duration and, over time, you will notice a change in the eighteen-hour-a-day fatigue you experienced before beginning your exercise routine.

Other benefits of walking include:

○ Two studies have found that brisk walking thirty minutes a day can postpone and even prevent the development of type 2 diabetes in people who are overweight.
○ It helps control high blood pressure.
○ It helps reduce LDL cholesterol and boost HDL cholesterol.
○ It reduces stress and tension.
○ It helps combat constipation, an extremely important consideration in view of the brain damage that can occur from toxins that are not moved quickly through the digestive system. Cirrhosis patients should have one or two bowel movements a day. Exercise will help you do that without laxatives.
○ It boosts your metabolic rate.
○ It helps prevent heart attacks and strokes. Just because you have cirrhosis does not mean you cannot get other life-threatening diseases. Cirrhosis patients should pay particular attention to their risk factors for heart disease and do what they can to reduce them.
○ It provides you with just the right amount of exposure to the sun, enough to meet your minimum requirements for vitamin D.

Another benefit of walking is the meditative peace of mind it offers. Individuals who have been walking on a regular basis for a year or more often find that it provides them with much-needed time for reflection, thereby opening the door to a better understanding of their disease.

TIPS FOR DAILY WALKS
Walking has become my favorite activity of the day. It makes me feel great, gives me a sense of accomplishment, and gives me time to think. On those occasions, especially during the holidays, when I have overeaten and

gained a pound or two, I have found that one or two walks are enough to get rid of the extra weight. Of course, my metabolism has something to do with that, but my body is so used to daily walks that they have become part of my body's metabolic formula.

Here are some tips to make your walks more pleasurable and beneficial:

○ Wear loose clothing that is appropriate to the amount of available sunlight.

○ Wear sunscreen, but be certain to read the warnings on the label.

○ If mosquitoes are a problem in your neighborhood, use extreme caution in using an insect repellent. Read the warnings on the label carefully. Personally, I think that DEET-based products are too toxic for cirrhosis patients, but if you are inclined to use a product with DEET, please talk to your doctor first.

○ When you walk during pollen season, wear a protective mask. Most of the medications used to reduce inflammation of the liver do so by suppressing the body's immune system. That means that your body will not be as effective as usual in combating the pollen that you inhale during your walks. If you don't protect yourself from pollen, you could get a sinus infection that could put unwanted stress on your liver.

○ Don't be intimidated by dogs on the loose. If that is a problem in your neighborhood, call the authorities. Don't stay inside and suffer in silence because you are afraid of offending your dog-owning neighbors. Meanwhile, purchase one of the spray repellents that vets sell.

○ Sometimes walking is more fun when you do it alone. Other times it is more fun when you do it with a friend or loved one. If you decide to cultivate a walking partner, make certain that it is not a reluctant volunteer. Nothing is worse than walking with someone who is constantly complaining that it is too hot or too cold or too wet or too early or too late!

Weight training

If you feel up to it, weight-bearing exercises can be a beneficial supplement to walking. Since all cirrhosis patients are at risk for osteoporosis, it is important to do what you can to offset the deterioration that will take place in your muscles and bones. Weight-bearing exercises increase muscle mass, which helps preserve bone strength.

You should consult with a fitness expert before starting weight training since your muscles, bones, and joints may have been weakened by your cirrhosis, in which case you will require a specialized workout program tailored to your needs.

If you have experienced complications of cirrhosis such as esophageal varices, you should not undertake weight training under any circumstances. Weight training could increase the pressure in your esophageal wall to the point where a rupture could take place and you could suffer a life-threatening hemorrhage.

IN A SENTENCE:

> *Regular exercise is one of the most important things you can do to help yourself stay healthy.*

learning

Obesity and Cirrhosis

THERE IS evidence that obesity is linked to cirrhosis through nonalcoholic liver disease. A 2003 study of eleven thousand patients published in *Gastroenterology* found that obesity increased the risk of death from cirrhosis in those who drank little or no alcohol, but not in alcoholics. Those findings are alarming for two reasons. First, because nonalcoholic fatty liver disease is the most common liver disease in the United States, and second, because the U.S. Centers for Disease Control reports that one-half of the U.S. adult population is overweight, with one-quarter of the population in the obese range.

Because of its links to cirrhosis and other serious diseases, obesity qualifies as a major health threat. From 1960 to 1994, the percentage of obese Americans jumped from 13 percent to 22.5 percent—and it has escalated to 25 percent in the years since then. Those figures are surprising to no one who has visited shopping malls, restaurants, or sporting events in recent years.

Researchers are at a loss to explain the weight explosion, but the major culprits seem to be decreased physical activity, increased social isolation, increased calorie consumption, and increased dining at restaurants that have boosted portion size in an effort to attract more customers.

Who says I'm obese?

In 1998 the National Heart, Lung, and Blood Institute released guidelines to assist health professionals in determining who is obese and who is not. According to the guidelines, there are three key measurements that can be used to determine obesity: body mass index (BMI), waist circumference, and a patient's risk factors for diseases and conditions associated with obesity. The guidelines define someone who is overweight as having a BMI of 25 to 20.9 and obesity as a BMI of 30 and above.

You can calculate your BMI by dividing your weight in kilograms by your height in meters squared. For example, a five-foot-six-inch man or woman who weighs 150 pounds will have a BMI of 24.2, just below the overweight category, while a man or woman of the same height who weighs 190 pounds will have a BMI of 30.7, enough to classify them as obese. By contrast, a five-foot person who weighs 150 pounds has a BMI of 29.45, enough to classify them as borderline obese.

A BMI of 30 is about thirty pounds overweight and is equal to about 220 pounds in a six-foot person and 186 pounds in someone who is five-foot-six. A waist circumference of over forty inches in men and over thirty-five inches in women indicates a significant health risk for those who have a BMI of 25 to 34.9.

For example, if you are a five-foot-six woman, weigh more than 150 pounds, and have a waistline larger than thirty-five inches—and if you drink little or no alcohol—you are at risk of developing nonalcoholic fatty liver disease that could develop into cirrhosis.

What is nonalcoholic fatty liver disease?

Fatty liver disease is a harmless condition that is characterized by fat deposits in the liver. It can be reversed and is not associated with any life-threatening liver diseases. However, nonalcoholic fatty liver disease (NAFLD) occurs when fatty liver progresses to an inflammation. It is not considered harmless at that point, since it can lead to cirrhosis or liver cancer. In an obese person, the entire liver may become made up of fat, which contrasts significantly with the liver of a healthy person of average weight, whose liver typically has 5 percent or less fat content.

NAFLD was named in 1980, when pathologists discovered that liver biopsies from people with fatty liver conditions that had led to inflammation and scarring were identical to those from people who had alcoholic liver disease, yet the former reported little or no alcohol consumption.

Individuals most likely to get NAFLD are those with type 2 diabetes, those with high levels of triglycerides in the blood, and those who meet the definition of being obese. Some researchers have concluded that it takes about ten years of obesity to put an individual at risk for developing cirrhosis. NAFLD is thought to account for about one-fourth of all the liver disease cases in the United States.

NAFLD is of great concern to health officials because of the skyrocketing obesity statistics. Since it takes ten years or more for cirrhosis to develop in NAFLD cases, and perhaps another ten to thirty years for it to reach the end stage, there is a fear that the health system will face liver disease cases of epidemic proportions in the years ahead.

What if I am obese and already have cirrhosis?

If you are an obese person with cirrhosis, it will be important for your doctor to determine whether your cirrhosis was caused by your excessive weight or whether your excessive weight was caused by your cirrhosis.

If you have had problems with your weight for a long time—ten years or longer—the odds are that your cirrhosis evolved from your obesity. If, on the other hand, your weight problems developed over a relatively short period of time (one to five years), they could be due to your disease. Fat is the most common reason for weight gain, but in cirrhosis patients, weight gain is sometimes due to fluid retention in the abdominal cavity (ascites), as well as in the feet and legs (edema). Medications taken by cirrhosis patients can also cause weight gain.

The normal reaction for an obese person who learns that they have cirrhosis is to lose the excess weight as soon as possible in an effort to improve their prognosis; but rapid weight loss at that point can be risky. It is recommended that obese cirrhosis patients ask their doctor to refer them to a weight-loss specialist who has experience with liver disease patients.

The worst thing you can do is to attempt a crash diet or ingest diet pills. Rapid weight loss is hard on a healthy liver; it can be devastating to a diseased liver. Rapid weight loss has the potential to push nonthreatening NAFLD into cirrhosis—and cirrhosis into complete liver failure. As far as diet pills are concerned, just remember that every pill you take has to be processed by the liver. The benefits of any weight loss you might achieve as the result of diet pills will likely be overshadowed by additional damage to your liver.

Is there anything I can do to safely lose weight?

There is more to weight gain than simply eating doughnuts by the case or living your life stretched out in front of the television as a couch potato. Excessive weight gain can be attributed to four factors, some of which occur simultaneously:

- ○ Physical inactivity
- ○ Increased calorie intake
- ○ Medical conditions
- ○ Isolation

Of the above-mentioned contributors to weight gain, it is isolation that offers the most potential for safe modification. Without a doubt, it is a major contributor to weight gain, once you exclude serious psychological or medical conditions. There are three types of isolation that most prominently contribute to weight gain (diet and exercise will be discussed in subsequent chapters):

Physical isolation. If you live and/or work alone, you are: (1) more likely to dine on fast food, take-out, or frozen dinners; (2) more likely not to have a significant other in your life, thus making you more likely to be unconcerned about your physical appearance; (3) more likely to experience health problems; and (4) more likely to suffer from chronic stress.

Emotional isolation. Emotional isolation almost always accompanies physical isolation, but it is possible to experience emotional isolation while living in a household with other individuals. It is characterized by a sense of separateness from others. It is often expressed by the following:
- ○ Excessive television viewing
- ○ Excessive Internet usage
- ○ Lack of sexual activity
- ○ Obsessions with pornography

Intellectual isolation. This type of isolation is sometimes expressed through obsessions with radical politics or various "lost causes." If you are obese and spend a great deal of time thinking about political and social issues, to the point of allowing your dedication to the "cause" to dominate your life, you may be a victim of your own good intentions and you may be compensating for your failure to turn your lost cause into a victory by stuffing yourself with food and sitting in front of the computer or television instead of exercising. Just remember that they don't call them "lost causes" for nothing.

Since these three types of isolation often are interrelated (for example, emotional isolation can lead to both physical and intellectual isolation), your best hope for losing weight may be to target your physical or emotional isolation and then to take a proactive approach to making meaningful changes in your life. Your best hope for doing that is to seek the help of a qualified therapist.

IN A SENTENCE:

If you are obese, losing weight is one of the most important things you can do to help treat your cirrhosis.

What Are the Complications of Cirrhosis?

THE DEVELOPMENT of complications in cirrhosis is a slow process. A person can have the disease for years, even decades, with no outward display of symptoms. That's because the damage that is being done occurs on a cell-by-cell basis, with each dying cell adding another brick in the mortar of scar tissue that builds within the liver.

Unless their disease is caused by an acute infection, accompanied by fever and vomiting, most cirrhosis patients have no idea that their liver is under attack. That is what is so insidious about cirrhosis: the fact that it suffers in silence for so many years.

However, there *is* a progression that the disease follows:

○ The first symptoms are fatigue, weakness, and exhaustion, followed by a loss of appetite with occasional nausea and weight loss.

○ As liver function declines, less protein, including albumin, is manufactured by the organ. The result is an accumulation of fluid in the legs (edema) and in the abdomen (ascites).

○ The patient begins to bruise easily, and cuts seem to take longer to heal, the result of a decrease in the proteins needed for blood clotting.

○ The patient develops jaundice and appears yellow.

○ The patient experiences intense itching, a result of bilirubin buildup in the skin.

○ Gallstones begin to form because the gallbladder is not receiving enough bile.

○ Men experience enlarged breasts (gynecomastia). This condition may be accompanied by shrunken testes.

○ The patient can develop skin problems such as red palms and small, spiderlike veins visible on the surface of the chest.

○ The patient develops decreased drug metabolism.

○ The patient develops "liver breath," a fruity, musty breath odor.

○ The patient can develop an enlarged liver and spleen.

○ Since one of the liver's functions is to filter toxins out of the blood, any damage done to the organ affects that process, allowing toxins to poison the brain. This process is called encephalopathy.

○ Varices are enlarged blood vessels (varicose veins) that form in the stomach and esophagus, the result of increased blood pressure due to blockage within the liver.

Edema and ascites

Your liver is the most clandestine organ in your body. It abhors publicity and avoids the limelight. It prefers to do its work "behind the scenes," and it resists attempts to strip away the mystery attached to its purpose. When it malfunctions, symptoms rarely manifest themselves in obvious ways, as is usually the case with other organs.

Edema and ascites are two exceptions to that rule, for they are two of the rare occasions when the liver allows its guard to drop. Edema occurs when there is fluid buildup in the legs. It is usually apparent in swollen ankles. *Ascites* is the term for the fluid buildup in the abdomen. The stomach will appear swollen and the patient will report having a bloated feeling.

Many men with "beer bellies" develop them because of years of consuming beer, with its high caloric content, but others develop protruding bellies because the alcohol in the beer has destroyed their liver function, caused cirrhosis, and allowed bodily fluids to build up in the abdominal cavity and in the ankles.

You can have cirrhosis for many years without displaying the symptoms of edema or ascites. When those two complications do appear, they are a cause for concern since it means that the scarring on the liver has progressed to the point where it is interfering with the manufacture of albumin.

Enlarged liver and spleen

The spleen lies below the diaphragm, to the left of the stomach and a little behind it. It is about five inches long and three to four inches wide. Soft and spongy, it acts as a repository for injured red blood cells and helps filter foreign substances from the blood.

When the body needs extra blood, the spleen squeezes out some of the blood it has stored and reinserts it into the bloodstream. Despite the important work it does, the spleen is only a helper for the other organs and glands and it can be removed from the body without any ill effects.

Doctors treating cirrhosis patients pay attention to the spleen because it provides indirect evidence of liver function. An enlarged spleen (**splenomegaly**) could mean that the patient has a viral disease such as hepatitis (about one third of hepatitis patients have enlarged spleens) or it could mean that the liver has been damaged by cirrhosis and has been asked to store the blood platelets that the liver can no longer process.

If your liver and spleen are enlarged, the condition will show up on your sonogram or CT scan. Additionally, your doctor will be able to determine whether either organ is enlarged by asking you to take a deep breath and then pressing firmly but gently below your rib cage on the right (for your liver) and below your rib cage on the left (for your spleen). Your doctor will also want to determine if there is any tenderness around your liver or spleen.

Enlarged male breasts (gynecomastia)

Gynecomastia can happen at any age. It is very common in newborn males, and is a result of exposure to the mother's hormones in breast milk. It can also occur during puberty, when teens are undergoing hormonal changes. When it occurs in adult males it almost always involves overeating, which results in an added layer of fat over the pectoral muscles, but there are certain diseases and conditions that can cause male breast enlargement, including kidney failure, tumors, adrenal cancer, liver disease, and side effects from drugs such as the androgen hormones taken by bodybuilders.

Of course, it is gynecomastia's relationship to liver disease with which we are most concerned. If cirrhosis causes gynecomastia, there will be other symptoms and complications present, though they might not be as apparent as the enlarged breasts.

Doctors and patients alike often overlook this symptom of cirrhosis because, for some, it is embarrassing to discuss. Seldom do male patients visit a doctor for the purpose of having their enlarged breasts evaluated. Most of the time, if the subject arises at all, it will be secondary to the stated purpose of the office visit.

Decreased drug metabolism

One early warning sign of cirrhosis is your body's inability to process medications, whether it is for high blood pressure, indigestion, infections, or any other condition. If you are being treated for a condition that requires medication and your doctor has to frequently change your dosage or change your medication entirely because you report side effects to everything she prescribes, it is time to ask for a liver evaluation.

It is your liver's job to metabolize the drugs that are put into your system. When it is unable to do its job, it will let you know by not metabolizing the drugs, thus making them appear ineffective.

If you have already been diagnosed with cirrhosis, do not be surprised if you develop reactions to drugs that once caused you no problems. Nor should you be surprised if your doctor has to go through several drugs to find one that your liver will successfully metabolize.

Glaucoma and cataracts

If you have been diagnosed with autoimmune hepatitis and you are taking prednisone as part of your treatment, you are at increased risk for both glaucoma and cataracts. Glaucoma is a disease that causes damage to the optic nerve and can lead to blindness. A cataract is a clouding of the eye's natural lens. Cataracts are a natural result of aging, but they also are caused by drugs such as prednisone.

I see an ophthalmologist every four months so that I can be checked for glaucoma and cataracts—and I recommend that you do the same.

Osteoporosis

Osteoporosis is the result of decreased bone mass and decreased bone density. It leads to a general weakening of your bones, which puts you at greater risk of bone fractures. Cirrhosis contributes to this condition by reducing your physical activity, reducing your muscle mass, and reducing your nutritional choices. Some medications, such as prednisone, can contribute to osteoporosis, so if you take prednisone you should talk to your doctor about the advisability of nutritional supplements.

Bleeding varices

Bleeding varices (varicose veins) in the esophagus or stomach are the most serious complication of cirrhosis. At some point in your treatment your doctor will want you to undergo an endoscopic examination so that she can determine: (1) whether you have developed varices; and (2) if they are present, whether they appear to be at risk of rupture. Many experts recommend that endoscopic examinations be performed every two or three years so that this development can be closely followed.

Varices are caused by the slow buildup of blood pressure in the liver, a condition known as portal hypertension. Since cirrhosis blocks blood flow through the liver, the veins compensate by enlarging and finding new routes around the organ so that blood can be returned to the heart. Varicose veins in the neck are called esophageal varices. Varicose veins in the stomach are called **gastric varices**.

Over time, the pressure in the varices builds to the point where the vein literally explodes, allowing bleeding into the throat or stomach. Early symptoms include weakness, lightheadedness, nausea, vomiting up blood or coffee-colored material, or bowel movements that are bloody or black.

If those symptoms are missed or ignored, the most ominous symptom—blood pouring into the throat—will be impossible to miss or ignore. When bleeding from varices occurs, it is a life-threatening medical emergency that requires immediate hospitalization. Fortunately, only one-third of people with cirrhosis ever get esophageal varices and, among those affected, only one-third ever experience bleeding.

Bleeding can be prevented by the use of medications that reduce pressure within the veins. Inderal is the drug most often used. If Inderal is not effective, the addition of a second drug, Imdur, often brings the desired results.

Encephalopathy

Encephalopathy is a brain dysfunction that is caused by the accumulation of toxic chemicals in the bloodstream, including but not limited to ammonia. Symptoms include irritability, depression, sleeplessness, personality changes, forgetfulness, slurred speech, tremors, and difficulty balancing. If not treated, encephalopathy can spiral out of control and result in the patient going into a coma.

If you have cirrhosis, pay close attention to any changes in your personality or lifestyle. Such changes, along with insomnia and irritability, may indicate that your brain is having a difficult time with unfiltered toxins from your liver. Another thing to watch for is constipation. Before you developed cirrhosis, it was no big deal. Now it is an important symptom that should not be ignored, since constipation allows toxins such as ammonia to accumulate in your intestines and potentially make their way to your brain, where they will interfere with your thought processes.

Liver cancer

Just when you thought nothing could be worse than a diagnosis of cirrhosis, you learn that the disease puts you at increased risk for another troublesome disease—liver cancer.

Your risk for developing liver cancer depends on the cause of your cirrhosis. If it is hepatitis C, you have a risk of between 1.5 to 6 percent *per year*, which means that ten years after being diagnosed you have a 15 to 60 percent chance of developing liver cancer. Men are more likely to get liver cancer than women, drinkers more likely than nondrinkers, and smokers more likely than nonsmokers.

If your cirrhosis is the result of alcohol abuse, you have a low to inter-mediate risk of developing liver cancer. If your cirrhosis is derived from nonalcoholic steatohepatitis (NASH), you have an intermediate risk. If your cirrhosis is caused by Wilson's disease, or autoimmune hepatitis, you have a very low risk of developing liver cancer.

learning

Coping with Complications When They Arise

*Having cirrhosis is such a waiting game.
I dreaded going to the doctor's office
because I feared news of a complication.
When it finally happened, it was in the form
of ascites, but it ceased to be a problem
when my doctor put me on a low-salt diet.*

—CHARLIE S.

NOT EVERYONE with cirrhosis experiences complications. You may go for many years without experiencing even the hint of a complication. But should any occur, it is to your advantage to know and understand the various treatments involved. Some of the treatments may seem overly invasive and radical to you (similar to what you would experience having a tooth pulled). Others will be noninvasive and almost inconsequential (similar to undergoing a chest X-ray). Your emotional and mental preparation will have a great deal to do with your response to those treatments.

Edema and ascites

Edema and ascites are two of the rare occasions when the liver allows its guard to drop. Edema occurs when there is fluid buildup in the legs. It is usually apparent by the appearance of swollen ankles. Ascites is the name for the fluid buildup in the abdomen. The stomach will appear swollen and the patient will report having a bloated feeling.

You can have cirrhosis for many years without displaying the symptoms of edema or ascites. When those two complications do appear, it is a cause for concern, since it means that the scarring on the liver has progressed to the point where it is interfering with the manufacture of albumin, with fluid buildup the most obvious result.

The primary treatments for this complication are salt restriction and diuretics. Your doctor will begin with suggestions on how to restrict your salt intake. If limiting your salt intake proves ineffective—and the swelling does not go away—your doctor may prescribe diuretics such as Aldactone or Lasix or Demadex. Diuretics sometimes cause severe muscle cramps, but they can be managed by lowering your salt intake and by taking magnesium supplements. Some diuretics (Aldactone, Inspra, Midamor, and Dyrenium) may make the potassium levels increase, while most diuretics make the potassium levels fall. Doctors try to balance the effects of potassium sparing with potassium wasting diuretics to optimize fluid loss and maintain potassium levels in the normal range. If you are already taking extra potassium, you should let your doctor know. Excessive potassium can be dangerous.

If the fluids in your abdominal cavity become infected, the condition is known as **spontaneous peritonitis**. It is characterized by abdominal pain, confusion, fever, and increased amounts of fluids. The treatment is intravenous antibiotics. The antibiotics most often used to prevent spontaneous peritonitis are fluoroquinolones (such as Cipro).

Sometimes salt restriction and diuretics are not enough to control the buildup of fluids. In that case, your doctor may want to place a needle into your abdominal cavity and withdraw the excess fluids using the suction created by manipulating the hypodermic. That process is called paracentesis.

If that treatment doesn't work, your doctor may want to do a procedure called a TIPS procedure (transjugular intrahepatic portal-systemic shunt). It involves the insertion of a needle through a vein in the jugular vein on the right side of the neck. The needle is passed into the hepatic vein and then advanced into the portal vein. This procedure creates a passageway for a catheter to be left in place between the hepatic and portal veins, decreasing the portal pressure and reducing the amount of ascetic fluid produced by the body. In years past, doctors used a procedure called a LeVeen or Denver shunt. It involved inserting a plastic tube into the abdominal cavity and a second plastic tube under the skin. The second tube was then tunneled up to the neck or chest, where it was inserted into a large vein. The purpose of this procedure was to allow the fluids in the abdominal cavity to drain into the bloodstream, where they could be more easily managed by the body. This procedure is rarely performed today.

Enlarged liver and spleen

Generally speaking, no treatment is necessary for a spleen enlarged due to cirrhosis. The problem is in the liver, not the spleen. Despite the important work it does, the spleen is only a helper for the other organs and glands. It can be removed from the body without any ill effects, but that is seldom done when the enlargement is due to cirrhosis.

Enlarged male breasts (gynecomastia)

There are medications that are effective in treating gynecomastia, but subjecting your liver to another drug will be the last thing your doctor will want to do. Your gynecomastia will likely subside when your liver inflammation subsides. Meanwhile, you probably have more serious problems to deal with.

Decreased drug metabolism

There is no treatment for decreased drug metabolism other than treating the cause of the cirrhosis.

Glaucoma and cataracts

There is no cure for glaucoma, but medication and surgery can often prevent further vision loss. Early detection is the key to stopping the progression of the disease.

Osteoporosis

Dr. Melissa Palmer recommends that all people with advanced chronic liver disease, especially women over the age of fifty, undergo bone-mineral-density testing to determine if they have osteoporosis. She recommends that people who are at high risk for osteoporosis (especially women with primary biliary cirrhosis) start taking Fosamax before bone loss occurs—and she recommends that liver patients who already have bone loss due to osteoporosis promptly take one of the three available medications for that condition: Fosamax, Didronel, or Actonel. However, patients with esophageal varices should avoid these medications, since the drugs are known to cause ulcers in the esophagus, a situation that could promote a life-threatening hemorrhage.

Bleeding varices

The Center for Abdominal Transplant at Tulane University Medical Center recommends the following treatments for individuals with bleeding varices:

Endoscopic therapy. An endoscope is a flexible lighted instrument that is inserted through the mouth for the purpose of examining the esophagus, stomach, and small intestine. The instrument allows the doctor to take one of two approaches to stop the bleeding. The first is called **sclerotherapy** and it involves the injection of a chemical solution into the varicose vein, made visible by the endoscope. The solution causes the blood inside the vein to clot, and if the procedure is performed repeatedly, it can make the vein disappear. The second approach is called **rubber band litigation.** It involves the placement of a rubber band on the varice, the purpose of which is to cause the same type of clotting prompted by sclerotherapy. Generally, three to five endoscopic sessions, at one- to four-week intervals, are required to make the veins disappear.

Surgical shunt. This is a procedure that diverts blood away from the liver, thereby lowering the pressure in the varicose veins in the esophagus. The procedure is usually used if sclerotherapy and rubber band litigation both prove ineffective at stopping the bleeding. Surgical shunts are usually effective, but they require major surgery, and some cirrhosis patients may not tolerate surgery well. Three potential complications of the surgical shunt are: (1) complete liver failure; (2) an increased risk of encephalopathy that could result in coma; and (3) serious problems with fluid retention. Furthermore, the procedure may interfere with a transplant surgeon's ability to perform a transplant. As a result, surgical shunts are used only for a carefully selected group of patients, whose primary problem from cirrhosis is bleeding.

TIPS shunt. If the surgical shunt doesn't work or is considered too risky, your doctor may install a TIPS shunt. TIPS is an abbreviation for transjugular intrahepatic portosystemic shunt. Don't be intimidated by the fancy name. It is a plastic tube that is inserted in the jugular vein and passed into the liver. A needle is inserted through the tube and a passage is created within the liver so that the main vein that brings blood into the liver can be connected to the main vein that carries blood from the liver to the heart. Once the passage has been created, a metal stent is inserted to keep the passage open. This procedure stops the bleeding in the esophagus by reducing the flow of blood into the varicose veins. The major advantage of a TIPS shunt is that it is less risky than a surgical shunt and it is less likely to interfere with future transplant needs.

TIPS shunts have also proven effective in patients with fluid retention that cannot be controlled by medication. Tulane University Medical Center estimates that 70 to 80 percent of the patients who undergo a TIPS shunt for management of ascites benefit from the procedure.

Encephalopathy

The treatment for encephalopathy focuses on: (1) antibiotics to kill the bacteria in the intestines that produces dangerous toxins such as ammonia (neomycin, Xifaxin, and Flagyl are the most commonly prescribed); (2) laxatives to prevent the buildup of ammonia in the intestines (lactulose is often prescribed); (3) limits on protein in the diet; and (4) the avoidance of medications that increase the brain's sensitivity to toxins—Valium, Demerol, Percocett, Darvocet, Xanax, Benadryl, Compazine, etc.

In the event that encephalopathy progresses to the stage where you are too sleepy to eat, doctors can insert a soft feeding tube through your nose and into your stomach to provide you with nutrients until a liver is available for transplant.

Liver cancer

Obviously, this is the nightmare complication of cirrhosis. However, if your doctor tells you that you have liver cancer, it is not the end of the world. As with everything else involving the liver, there are options, which we will discuss in more detail in a subsequent chapter devoted entirely to that subject (Month 6).

IN A SENTENCE:

> *If you experience complications, no matter how frightening, know that your doctor has a plan and a backup to that plan to cover every possibility.*

living

Dealing with Depression

*I had never been depressed a day in my life
until I was told I had cirrhosis. After that everything
changed and, no matter what I did, I could not
shake the sadness that hung over me like a dark cloud.*

—ELAINE Z.

SOMETIMES DEPRESSION is an illness. Other times
it is a perfectly natural reaction to an unnatural life situation
that is cloaked in stress or tragedy. Whether it is an illness or a
natural reaction to life's misfortunes, depression has a profound
effect on the human body and it will make your recovery from
cirrhosis difficult if you succumb to it.

Yes, you heard me correctly—succumb! My experience as a
social worker has led me to believe that it is within everyone's
power to reject depression. I do not believe that depression is
a mysterious chemical brew in the brain over which we have no
control, unless, of course, it is a direct result of the side effects
that sometimes accompany many prescription drugs.

Each year, more than nineteen million Americans age eighteen and over suffer from a depressive illness. It is the leading
cause of disability in the United States, according to a recent
study by the World Health Organization and Harvard University. Nearly twice as many women as men are affected by the

illness. Just how many of those nineteen million are being treated for hepatitis or cirrhosis is unknown, but research has shown that up to 30 percent of patients being treated for hepatitis C suffer from depression.

If you have been diagnosed with hepatitis or cirrhosis—or any other life-threatening illness—you are at risk for depression.

What are the symptoms of depression?

You are probably already aware of the obvious symptoms of depression: a deep feeling of despair, a vague sense of having the blues—a belief that the world as you know it is coming to an end. But those "obvious" symptoms are often fleeting and they may be masked by more important symptoms that reveal more about your actual state of mind:

- ○ Eating problems—either eating too much or too little
- ○ Sleeping problems
- ○ Inability to concentrate
- ○ Lack of energy
- ○ Feelings of worthlessness
- ○ Irritability
- ○ Unexplained flashes of anger
- ○ Thoughts of death

What is the cause of my depression?

You may have noticed that many of the symptoms of depression are similar to the manifestations of cirrhosis. For that reason, it is important that you go over any depression-related symptoms with your doctor so that she can help you decide which are related to the complications of your cirrhosis and which are related to preexisting emotional issues.

For example, sleeping problems can be due to side effects from drugs such as prednisone or they can be due to changes in your brain due to encephalopathy. Interferon, which is used to treat hepatitis C patients, is known to cause mood swings and irritability. Other medications cause similar symptoms. Some thyroid disorders caused by cirrhosis-related problems can cause symptoms identical to depression. Likewise, anemia caused by liver malfunction can produce symptoms similar to depression.

Whether your depression is related to your cirrhosis and its treatment, or to your emotional reaction to having cirrhosis, you need to deal with it before it affects your recovery in a negative manner.

If your doctor determines that your depression is the result of your treatment, or a complication of your disease, she will probably modify your medication and her treatment of the complication. If your doctor determines that your depression is the result of emotional issues, she will probably recommend that you see a therapist.

Your first task is to determine when the depression began. Ask yourself the following questions:

○ Do you have a history of depression? That is, did you suffer from depression before you learned you have cirrhosis? If so, when did it begin? Were you depressed as a child? As an adolescent? As a young adult? Have you ever been prescribed medication for depression? Have you ever talked to a therapist about your depression? Are you currently on medication for depression?

○ Did your depression begin when you were diagnosed with hepatitis or cirrhosis? Has it lasted longer than a few weeks? Are you taking medication for hepatitis or cirrhosis? Have you ever felt depressed on previous occasions when confronted with bad news?

Why am I depressed?

It's possible that your depression may be an emotional reaction to your cirrhosis diagnosis or a side effect from your treatment. However, if you feel your depression began long before your diagnosis, you might first re-examine your life, beginning with your childhood. Did you experience any health-related traumas as a child? Did you lose a parent to death or divorce? Were you raised by a single parent? Were you abused as a child? Were you able to make friends as a child? Did you have to change schools often because your parent or parents were relocated because of their jobs? If you answered yes to any of the above, you have a childhood foundation for depression as an adult.

Research tells us that the following children are more likely to experience depression as adults:

- ○ Children raised by a single parent
- ○ Children who were abused
- ○ Children who changed schools often
- ○ Children who lost a parent to divorce or death
- ○ Children who underwent major surgery and suffered complications
- ○ Children who were unable to bond with their parents
- ○ Adopted children

Children who carry any of the above issues with them into adolescence are likely to undergo depression as teens, especially if any of the above issues prevents them from adequately socializing with their peers. Issues that began as childhood emotional injuries resulting from issues such as abuse or abandonment will be magnified in adolescence and characterized by unexplained anger and hostility.

If the issues are not resolved in adolescence, they will be carried into adulthood, where they will be characterized by an inability to sustain long-term romantic relationships, poor self-image, a dependency on alcohol or drugs, a tendency to choose life partners who are abusive, and the list goes on and on.

What Can I Do about My Depression?

The experts recommend a three-step approach to dealing with your depression.

Step one: Work with your doctor to find out if it is related to your disease and/or its treatment. The problem may be remedied by modifying your medication or choosing alternative treatment methods. For example, the symptoms associated with encephalopathy sometimes mimic the symptoms of depression. Treatment of the encephalopathy may help the depressive symptoms. Give your doctor an opportunity to identify and treat disease-related causes of your depression before you seek the services of a therapist.

Step two: Work with a therapist, either a social worker or a psychologist, who is experienced with problems related to disease. There are many possible causes for your depression, but you have to identify them before you can treat them. Your therapist's first goal will be to establish how long you have been depressed. The second goal will be to identify the possible causes of your depression. Among the possibilities are:

○ Alcoholism (alcohol is a depressant)
○ Childhood trauma (incest, sexual abuse, childhood diseases, etc.)
○ Adult trauma (rape, sexual abuse, numerous failed relationships)
○ Obesity. If you were overweight as a child, you should reexamine your childhood. Did you play alone as a child? Do you feel you had meaningful childhood relationships? And, perhaps most important of all, did you watch a lot of television? Recent studies have indicated that children consume about 25 percent of their daily food in front of the television, a blueprint for obesity. If your weight gain occurred as an adult, were there traumatic experiences that preceded it, such as the death of a loved one or the failure of a romantic relationship? Look back over your life.
○ Isolation (as discussed earlier in the book, emotional, physical, and intellectual isolation can contribute to depression).

Step three: Based on the successful completion of steps one and two, you should deal with the problems that caused your depression. You may argue that it was your depression that caused your alcoholism or your obesity or your sense of isolation in the first place. Even if that is true, you must turn loose the past so that you can deal with the present and the future. That means accepting alcoholism and obesity and isolation as causes of your depression as presently defined.

Your doctor will probably know a good therapist for you to see about your depression. If not, depending on your comfort level, you might want to ask your friends if they know a therapist they would recommend. Another option would be to contact the state office for the American Psychological Association and ask to speak to the person who handles their referral service.

What you do not want to do is pick a psychologist or social worker at random, since many specialize in areas that would have no bearing on your situation (children, work-related problems, seniors, etc.). For more information about therapists, see the Living section in Month 2.

IN A SENTENCE:

Depression is something that you can successfully deal with.

learning

What Does Sleep Have to Do with It?

> It bothers me that I can't seem to sleep anymore.
> It makes me irritable and when that happens
> I feel guilty. I spend more time worrying about that
> than I do worrying about my cirrhosis.
>
> —ASHLEY B.

ONE OF the first symptoms of your cirrhosis was probably sleepiness and fatigue—and, if you are like everyone else, you ignored that symptom and attributed it to staying up too late the night before, or insomnia due to too much coffee, or the rainstorm that came through after midnight and awakened you.

Since sleep issues are a possible indicator of problems with your liver, they are also an indicator of the progress you are making in your treatment. If you are able to sleep through the night—and get eight hours of sleep—it is a good indication that you are doing everything correctly and your treatment is headed in the right direction.

If, on the other hand, you are experiencing sleep problems, it is an indication that you need to make changes in your life. Sleep is every bit as important as exercise, diet, and medication in your recovery.

How much sleep do you need?

In a 2003 study, researchers at the University of Pennsylvania found that subjects who slept four to six hours a night for fourteen consecutive nights showed significant deficits in cognitive performance equivalent to going without sleep for up to three days in a row. Amazingly, the subjects in the study reported feeling only slightly sleepy. They were totally unaware of how impaired they were from lack of sleep.

In study after study, researchers have found that eights hours of sleep each night is required to maintain good health. If you get less than that, you may feel fine, like the subjects in the University of Pennsylvania study, but there is a lot more to good health than what is visible on the surface and if you have liver disease you can be certain that a lack of sleep is causing problems that may take weeks or months to become evident.

Is sleep an issue in your life?

Here are a few questions you can ask yourself to determine whether sleep, or rather the lack of it, is an issue in your life:

- O Do you fall asleep while you are sitting in a chair watching television or reading?
- O Do you fall asleep when you are a passenger in a car?
- O As a driver, have you ever fallen asleep while stopped at a traffic light?
- O Have you ever fallen asleep while talking on the telephone?
- O Have you ever fallen asleep while sitting and talking to someone?
- O Have you ever fallen asleep while attending a meeting or watching a movie?
- O Do you get sleepy at a certain time each afternoon?

If you answered yes to any of the above questions, sleep is clearly an issue in your life. Before you decide what to do about it, you need to examine the possible causes of your sleeping difficulties. Here are some of the possibilities:

Medication. Are you taking prednisone or interferon? Both drugs are known to cause sleeping problems. If you did not have sleeping problems before you started the medication, the odds are good that the medication is at fault. It is highly unlikely that your doctor will want to modify your medication because of sleep problems, especially not if the medicine is bringing about improvements in your cirrhosis or hepatitis.

Encephalopathy. Sleep disorders may be a symptom of encephalopathy, so it is important that you report any sleeping problems to your doctor. Self-treatment with sleeping medications is definitely to be avoided since it could make the problem worse.

Bad sleeping habits. Are you staying up too late at night? Do you take naps of an hour or longer during the day? Do you read or watch television in bed? Do you drink coffee or tea or soft drinks with caffeine in the evenings? The solution to your sleep problems may lie in changing your sleeping habits.

Anxiety over your illness. If you have negative thoughts throughout the day about your illness, especially if you are fearful of dying, those fears will accumulate and present themselves to you for resolution at bedtime. That's because your subconscious mind knows that this is your last opportunity to resolve those issues before going to sleep, and it will do its best to keep you awake. This is a situation in which a therapist would be of great help. If you are religious, your minister, priest, or rabbi may be able to allay your fears to the point where you can resume more normal sleep patterns.

Relationship problems. If you are having problems with your partner, you may resist going to bed as a way of resisting intimacy with your partner. Your sleep problems may have nothing to do with your cirrhosis. You may lie awake for hours experiencing anxiety over your inability or unwillingness to be intimate with your partner. Guilt is a notorious hindrance to sleep. If you are having relationship problems, I recommend that you talk to a therapist before making your sleep problems your doctor's responsibility.

Sleep-related illnesses. It is possible that you may have developed a condition known as irregular sleep-wake rhythm, one of several circadian rhythm disorders. People who have this sleep disorder often get eight hours of sleep over a twenty-four-hour period, but they get it in increments during the day and night in patterns that are not predictable. If your sleep problems began with your diagnosis of cirrhosis, or began shortly after you started taking prednisone or interferon, I would not be too quick to attribute them to a condition such as irregular sleep-wake rhythm disorder. If you follow all the tips in this chapter and still can't get a handle on a decent sleep pattern, then you might want to talk to your doctor about medical conditions unrelated to your cirrhosis.

It could be age related. If you are past fifty, you must consider the possibility that your sleep problems may be influenced by aging. Healthy people in their twenties and thirties usually fall asleep quickly and sleep through the night without awakening. But as people enter their forties and fifties, they are more likely to take longer to fall asleep and are more likely to be awakened by a barking dog or a windy rainstorm.

By the time a person is in their fifties and their hair has begun to gray and their vision has become blurry, they are more likely to toss and turn before going to sleep, and they are more likely to get up during the night to go to the bathroom. It is a natural part of the aging process that cannot be blamed on your cirrhosis. The only solution is to get younger. If you are able to do that, we need to talk.

Tips for getting a good night's sleep

- ❍ Eliminate caffeine from your diet.
- ❍ Do not exercise within six hours of your bedtime.
- ❍ Establish a bedtime and stick to it.
- ❍ Don't eat before going to bed.
- ❍ Don't watch television, read, write, or talk on the telephone while in bed.
- ❍ Get up at the same time each morning.
- ❍ If something upsets you shortly before bedtime, break your schedule and read a book or watch television for an hour or so before going to bed—just don't do it while in bed.
- ❍ Place a dim light in your bedroom that you can turn off when you go to bed. The last thing you want to do is turn on a bright light in your bedroom. You want your bedroom to be dark and slightly cool.

IN A SENTENCE:

A good night's sleep is worth fighting for, so knock yourself out.

What If I Get Liver Cancer?

*One of the first things my doctor told me
was that he wanted me to be proactive
in my efforts to avoid liver cancer.
It makes me feel better to know that
I have some control over that.*

—CONSTANCE T.

WHEN YOU were told that you had cirrhosis, you probably thought that there could not possibly be any more ominous news in your future. But once the shock of the diagnosis wore off, along came the news that having cirrhosis makes it more likely that you will develop liver cancer.

The bad news is that only 5 percent of patients diagnosed with liver cancer survive five years. But the good news is that the odds are still very much in your favor to avoid the disease, provided you take a proactive approach to preventing it.

There are many types of liver cancer, some of which originate in the liver and others that spread to the liver from other cancer sites. However, in this chapter I will focus on a cirrhosis-related primary liver cancer called **hepatocellular carcinoma**. You may never have heard of it, but it is one of the most common cancers in the world, with up to one million cases reported each year. It is the fifth most common cancer in men and the ninth most common cancer in women.

Your risk for this cancer is related to the cause of your cirrhosis. You are at greatest risk if your cirrhosis is due to:

○ Hemochromatosis
○ Alpha 1-antitrypsin deficiency
○ Hepatitis B and C
○ Alcoholic cirrhosis

You are at an intermediate risk for liver cancer if your cirrhosis is due to:

○ NASH

You are at lowest risk for liver cancer if your cirrhosis is due to:

○ Autoimmune hepatitis
○ Primary biliary cirrhosis

Patients with cirrhosis due to hepatitis C are typically scrutinized more closely for cancer by doctors because of the strong correlation that exists between the two diseases. If you have cirrhosis due to hepatitis C, your risk of developing liver cancer ranges between 1.5 to 6 percent per year. That means that five years after being diagnosed, your chances of developing liver cancer are somewhere between 7.5 and 30 percent—and ten years after being diagnosed, your chances are 15 to 60 percent. You can improve those odds by avoiding the threats listed in the following section.

Cancer threats to cirrhosis patients

Cirrhosis patients should be concerned about developing cancer from outside sources, since the scarring that has taken place inside your liver has made it impossible for the organ to protect you with the efficiency for which it was designed.

As you've learned, every vitamin, mineral, virus, chemical, bacterium, etc. that enters your body has to pass through your liver at some point to be filtered and metabolized. If your liver is scarred with dead tissue, the flow that normally takes place will be blocked, thus allowing toxins to build up in healthy tissue and subjecting individual cells to cancerous changes.

As a cirrhosis patient, there are four carcinogens that should concern you:

Alcohol. It is not a direct cause of cancer, but it can speed up the progression of cancer when combined with other carcinogens. Statistically speaking, 10 percent of patients with alcoholic cirrhosis will develop liver cancer in their lifetime. Alcoholic cirrhosis patients who stop drinking live, on average, ten years longer than those who continue to drink. One group of researchers examined autopsy reports on people who had alcoholic cirrhosis, and they found the presence of cancer in 55 percent of the cases.

Cigarette smoke. Various studies have found cigarette smoke a risk factor in the development of liver cancer, even in patients who did not have hepatitis. There is much to be learned about the relationship between cigarette smoke and liver cancer, but enough is known to recommend that cirrhosis patients not use tobacco products or subject themselves to secondhand cigarette smoke.

Aflatoxin. *Aspergillus flavus* is a fungus that grows in foods such as peanuts, soybeans, corn, and rice in hot, humid conditions for long periods of time. A by-product of the fungus is a carcinogen called **aflatoxin**. In Asian and African countries where peanuts and rice are sometimes stored in hot, humid conditions, the correlation between aflatoxin and liver cancer is very high.

American food processors are said to remove 90 percent of the mold in their products during the drying process, but that still leaves 10 percent to make its way into food products. A new danger to Americans may be the increased amount of food produced and processed outside the country, where inspection standards are often lax.

Should cirrhosis patients eat peanut butter, corn, soybeans, and rice?

It would be difficult to eliminate those foods entirely from your diet. However, there are steps you can take to put the odds more in your favor. For example, I recommend that you not eat any of the aflatoxin-friendly foods that are produced and processed outside the country. Read the labels. Look for foods with American addresses. If an American company describes itself as the distributor and does not provide an American address where the food was produced or processed, you can be fairly certain that the food was imported. You also should closely examine at-risk food products for discoloration, or nuts or grains that are stuck together.

Drugs, especially anabolic steroids, and oral contraceptives. People who take anabolic steroids as part of a muscle-building program are at increased risk of developing liver cancer. Cirrhosis patients who use the drugs should stop immediately. There is also evidence that women who use oral contraceptives for eight years or longer have an increased risk of liver cancer. Female cirrhosis patients who take oral contraceptives should find alternate means of birth control.

How is liver cancer diagnosed?

Diagnosing liver cancer can present a challenge for your doctor. Your doctor's main tools are a blood test called the AFP (alpha-fetoprotein) and the usual assortment of imaging devices—ultrasound, CT, and MR. The problem with the blood test is that only about one-third of patients with liver cancer have very high levels of AFP. That means that two-thirds of them have normal or low readings. To complicate the matter, many patients with hepatitis B or C have high AFP readings with no evidence of cancer. The test would appear to be useful only if your readings change from low or normal to high—and you are not being treated for hepatitis B or C. In that case, your doctor would probably want you to undergo a scan to see if any changes have taken place inside your liver.

You would think that would be a simple matter, but it is not. CT scans, MRs, and ultrasounds have an excellent track record for finding tumors, with one exception—liver tumors in cirrhosis patients are very difficult for the scans to identify because of the scarring and nodules caused by the cirrhosis.

A "clean" CT, MR, or ultrasound does not mean that your liver is free of cancer. It merely means that the scans did not detect cancer. The cancer may be there, lurking behind the scarring between two benign nodules. To be fair to the radiologists who read the scans, skilled surgeons often have a difficult time visually separating cancerous nodules from benign nodules in the liver.

That is why this disease is a challenge for your doctor. She can do everything right—she can give you the AFP blood test, an assortment of scans—and still miss the tumor. Even the act of screening you for cancer presents your doctor with various dilemmas. First, she must decide how often to screen you. The blood test poses no health risk to you, but the CT scan does, since it puts you at risk for radiation exposure and makes you vulnerable to a life-threatening allergic reaction to the iodine dye used in the procedure. Ultrasounds are the safest screening devices that can be used.

Once your doctor decides what kind of screening she is going to use with you, she must decide how often to do it. Intervals of six months to one year are typical. Generally, doctors screen cirrhosis patients for cancer only if they feel that they are good candidates for transplantation or surgical removal of a tumor.

How is liver cancer treated?

For liver cancer to be treatable in cirrhosis patients, the tumor must be smaller than two inches in diameter. Patients with tumors greater than two inches in diameter, or with multiple tumors (more than three), or with an aggressive tumor, are not candidates for surgery since a tumor larger than two inches may already have spread to other organs; nor are such patients candidates for transplantation. "However, sometimes even large tumors do not spread until the very late stages of disease," explains Dr. Regenstein. "In other cases, a small tumor may metastasize early. It really depends more on what we call the biologic behavior of the individual tumor."

Patients who have tumors that are considered treatable have several options:

Surgical removal of the tumor. This is usually the best option for liver cancer patients who do not have cirrhosis, but if cirrhosis is present, the odds for successful treatment are greatly lowered because even if the tumor is completely removed, the remaining liver tissue is usually too damaged after surgery to function. The success rate for surgery is low—only 10 to 20 percent of all hepatocellular carcinoma surgeries succeed in entirely removing all the cancerous tissue. If the surgery is not successful, according to the American Liver Foundation, the disease is often fatal within three to six months.

Abalation procedures (percutaneous alcohol injection, radiofrequency ablation [RFA] and cryoablation). These therapies work best on small tumors. The larger the tumor, the more difficult it becomes to completely destroy all the remaining tumor cells. Percutaneous alcohol injection involves the injection of a needle into the liver under the guidance of an ultrasound. The needle is placed directly into the tumor, and alcohol is fed into the tumor through the needle. The goal is for the alcohol to kill the cancer cells. This procedure reports high success rates for patients without cirrhosis, but the rates are much lower when advanced cirrhosis is present.

Tumor embolization. This procedure deliberately mimics what happens when a person has a heart attack due to a blood clot, only in this instance the goal is to create a blood clot in the artery that leads to the liver in the belief that clogging the artery will shut off the blood supply to the cancer cells and kill them. It is usually combined with chemotherapy. This treatment is usually reserved for patients who are not candidates for surgery or patients with tumors who are awaiting transplant. "Cirrhotic patients often will not tolerate removal of the tumor," says Dr. Regenstein. "They develop liver failure. In a normal liver you can remove up to 80 percent and it will grow back. In a cirrhotic liver, even removal of a small amount may lead to liver failure because the liver is not able to regenerate." Ablation and chemotherapy may be done prior to transplant to keep the tumors from enlarging and spreading while a patient waits for a donor liver.

Transplantation. To be a candidate for a successful transplant, your tumor needs to be smaller than two inches in diameter and not part of a tumor cluster. It is also important that your tumor not have spread to tissue beyond the liver.

If you are concerned about liver cancer, the best thing you can do is to adopt behavior that will help prevent cancer from ever developing in your liver. Among the things you can do to increase your odds:

○ Stop drinking and smoking, and avoid people who do either.
○ If you have viral hepatitis, undergo treatment; if you do not have viral hepatitis, be certain that you are vaccinated against hepatitis B and C.

○ If you are an IV drug user, stop.
○ Practice safe sex, using a condom—even if it is with a partner you have known for a long time.
○ Exercise and maintain a healthy diet designed to boost your immune system.
○ Avoid stress.
○ Avoid people with negative attitudes toward life.

IN A SENTENCE:

> *If you have cirrhosis and you are concerned about liver cancer, leave as little to chance as possible by being proactive about cancer prevention.*

learning

Children with Cirrhosis

I look at my poor baby,
and all I can do is cry.
It just seems so unfair.

—ALICE P.

FOR MOST parents, it comes as a shock that their children can get cirrhosis, but it is a disease that does not discriminate on the basis of age. It can affect people at any age, from infancy through old age. Although the percentage of children who get cirrhosis is quite small compared to adults, statistics are no comfort to the parents of a child who has the disease.

Billy Jr. was one month old when the doctor told Gretchen and Billy that he had hepatitis B. Gretchen and Billy were stunned by the news. They both underwent blood tests and learned that Gretchen had the disease. The doctor explained that she had passed the disease on to their son. The doctor said that he did not know how Gretchen had gotten hepatitis, but he added that that was not unusual since it is much easier to diagnosis the disease than it is to determine its cause. Thirty percent of the time, doctors are unable to trace the origins of the disease in a patient.

The doctor put Billy Jr. on antiviral medication and was pleased with his progress for the next several months. However,

when Billy Jr. went to the doctor for his one-year checkup, he was diagnosed with cirrhosis. Gretchen and Billy were heartbroken at first, but then
the doctor explained his treatment plan, and they felt better about Billy Jr.'s
prognosis.

As the years went by, and Billy Jr. grew from being a toddler to a pre-
schooler, it became obvious to Gretchen and Billy that cirrhosis was a disease with which they could live. They closely watched Billy Jr.'s diet and
they monitored his medications and made certain each year that he was
vaccinated against flu and pneumonia.

By the time Billy Jr. entered high school, it was clear that the cirrhosis
had been contained and was no longer spreading throughout his liver.
Shortly after his seventeenth birthday, a biopsy revealed that portions of his
previously scarred liver had been replaced by healthy tissue.

Major causes of cirrhosis in children

Hepatitis. When newborns or young children are infected with hepatitis B, their immune systems are not strong enough to kill the disease. As a result, about 90 percent of babies born with hepatitis B
develop a chronic case of the disease. A 1990 study undertaken by
French doctors looked at ninety-two children with chronic hepatitis
B. The doctors found that 32 percent of the children had cirrhosis.
In six of the children, cirrhosis was diagnosed within the first twelve
months of the onset of the disease.

Dr. Howard J. Worman is generally optimistic about the prognosis for children with chronic hepatitis B. Says Worman: "These parents often think that it is the end of the world for their child.
However, the parents should realize that most children with liver disease will do well. Most importantly, as for adults, they should plan for
their children to lead full and normal lives and remember that liver
transplantation is an 'insurance policy' if needed."

Hepatitis C has been known to be transferred from mother to
child, but this is not a common occurrence and takes place less than
7 percent of the time. However, the likelihood of transmission to the
child is increased if the mother also has HIV. In those instances
where infants test positive for hepatitis C, their immune systems are
likely to throw off the disease by age two.

Alpha 1-Antitrypsin deficiency. This is a hereditary disorder in which the absence of the enzyme alpha 1-antitrypsin causes liver disease. About 25 percent of children with this deficiency develop cirrhosis and die before the age of twelve. About 25 percent die by age twenty. The remaining 50 percent survive into adulthood with only minor problems. The only fully successful treatment is liver transplantation. This disease is rare in adults, but when it occurs it can lead to liver cancer.

Alcoholic liver disease. Women with this disease are usually infertile, but if they do become pregnant and continue to drink during their pregnancy, they put their infants at risk for **fetal alcohol syndrome**, a condition that could give their infants cirrhosis.

Wilson's disease. This is an inherited disease that, as mentioned above, is characterized by an accumulation of copper in the liver. A healthy liver will excrete the copper that enters the body, but for reasons that are not clearly understood, children with recessive genes for this disease accumulate life-threatening levels of copper in their livers. Most patients have no family history of the disease, but it is known to be transmitted from generation to generation through abnormal genes. The median age for this disease is eight to twenty years. Eventually, all children with this disease will develop cirrhosis.

Autoimmune hepatitis. This disease can occur in children as early as infancy, but most cases (70 percent) are found in female patients between the ages of fifteen and forty. Children with this disease are treated with the same prednisone/azathioprine protocol as adults— and with equally encouraging results. In one out of every three children, treatment can eventually be stopped.

Biliary atresia. This is the most common cause of cirrhosis in infants. It occurs because the child's bile ducts are absent or somehow injured, causing the bile to back up in the liver. The first symptoms, which usually include jaundice and dark urine, appear two to eight weeks after birth. The disease affects girls more than boys, and it affects Asians and African-Americans more than Caucasians.

There are no medications for the treatment of this disease, but there are two procedures that are used to treat the disease: first, the **Kasai procedure** is an operation in which the damaged ducts are replaced with a piece of the infant's intestine that is shaped to form a new duct that will allow bile to flow from the liver into the intestine. If the surgeon is experienced in the procedure, it is successful in 60 to 85 percent of cases. However, it is not a cure and only allows the child to enjoy good health for several years. Half of children who undergo the procedure will need a transplant by the time they are five years of age. Second, the other treatment option is a liver transplant. Since 85 percent of children who are diagnosed with biliary atresia will need a liver transplant by the time they are twenty, doctors usually prepare parents for that eventuality many years in advance.

Steatohepatitis/obesity. This is the stage of nonalcoholic fatty liver disease (NAFLD) that is characterized by liver inflammation. It can affect children at any age, but it occurs with greatest frequency during adolescence among obese children. The United States' obesity epidemic is relatively new, and research data is only now beginning to surface, but it is clear that obese children are at considerable risk for developing cirrhosis as a result of NASH. The most effective treatment for steatohepatitis is weight reduction. Left untreated, it can progress to cirrhosis, liver failure, and liver cancer. Texas Children's Hospital, which treats children with steatohepatitis, reports that patients who lose more than 10 percent of their body weight experience significant improvement.

Cystic fibrosis. Up to 40 percent of patients with cystic fibrosis develop cirrhosis and to date no therapeutic regimen has proven effective in preventing the progression of the disease. Symptoms can occur at any age, but the probability of symptoms increases with age until adolescence. Both single-liver and triple-organ (heart, lung, and liver) transplants have been performed on cystic fibrosis patients, but there is not enough available data for predictive analysis.

How to protect children from cirrhosis

Most children who have cirrhosis did not acquire it because of any ill-advised behavior on their part, and most of the time, parents are helpless to prevent it. However, there are behavior-related and lifestyle conditions in which children can get cirrhosis where parents can make a difference:

○ Parents have it within their power to protect their present and future children from hepatitis B by not engaging in risky behavior that will put their children at risk. That means saying no to IV drug use and unprotected sex, and seeking help for alcoholism.

○ Parents should make certain that obese children are enrolled in weight-reduction programs. Losing 10 percent of their weight could be lifesaving.

○ Parents should make certain that the child is vaccinated against hepatitis B. More and more infants are being routinely vaccinated against this disease.

IN A SENTENCE:

Children are also vulnerable to cirrhosis, but in some cases parents can decrease their risk by avoiding unsafe lifestyle choices.

HALF-YEAR MILESTONE

What You Should Have Done by Now

○ YOU HAVE SOUGHT OUT OTHER CIRRHOSIS PATIENTS.

○ YOU HAVE LEARNED THE COMPLICATIONS THAT CAN ARISE WITH YOUR DISEASE—AND HOW THOSE COMPLICATIONS ARE TREATED.

○ YOU HAVE STARTED AN EXERCISE PROGRAM.

○ YOU HAVE IDENTIFIED A DIET THAT IS RIGHT FOR YOU.

○ YOUR DOCTOR HAS DEVISED A TREATMENT PLAN TAILORED TO YOUR SPECIFIC NEEDS.

○ YOU HAVE LEARNED HOW TO DEAL WITH DEPRESSION.

○ YOU SLEEP EIGHT HOURS A NIGHT.

○ YOU HAVE LEARNED HOW TO BE ALERT TO LIVER CANCER.

Senior Citizens with Cirrhosis

People give me the oddest looks
when I tell them that I have cirrhosis.
When I see those looks, I always say,
"Don't worry about it—I've had worse!"

—HENRY G.

THANKS TO today's medical advances, we have the benefit of living longer than previous generations, and no one would argue that increased life expectancy is not a good thing. However, when it comes to cirrhosis, longevity presents a different set of challenges for seniors than those faced by younger patients.

As the healthy liver ages, it changes in ways that sometimes make treatment for liver disease more difficult. Its volume naturally decreases with age (less liver means less function). There is a decrease in blood flow through the liver. And the liver becomes less efficient at regenerating new tissue.

Andrew M. was seventy years old when he was diagnosed with cirrhosis. He had no overt symptoms and was diagnosed only because routine blood work showed an elevation in his liver enzymes. Andrew's doctor, who had known him for only five years, was perplexed at first, because he knew his patient to be a nondrinker and the tests for hepatitis all came back negative.

"You don't drink, do you?" asked the doctor.

"No, I don't," answered Andrew.

Andrew didn't bother to tell his doctor that he had been a heavy drinker for thirty years before stopping at the age of sixty. It was simply a part of his life that he didn't want to talk about. He didn't drink *now*, and to his way of thinking, that was what was important.

Andrew's doctor diagnosed him with cryptogenic cirrhosis, meaning there was no apparent cause. He put Andrew on vitamins and explained that he wanted to monitor the progress of his disease with blood tests and ultrasound for several months in the hopes of learning more about the cause of his cirrhosis. That was fine with Andrew. He had no obvious symptoms of cirrhosis and he was more concerned about the heart attack he had had five years earlier. Whenever he had fleeting thoughts about death, that was what he thought about—clutching his chest and dropping to the ground. Cirrhosis was a mystery to him. He didn't know enough about the disease to fear its consequences.

Andrew reported to his doctor on a regular basis for a year, with no noticeable changes in his health. Then one day, seemingly out of the blue, his doctor told him that he had bad news: the ultrasound had indicated a mass in his liver. Andrew had liver cancer. Fortunately, the tumor was less than an inch in diameter and was not particularly aggressive. Andrew was evaluated for a transplant and, one year later, at the age of seventy-two, he received a new liver—surgery that was made possible because his tumor had grown only about a half inch during the twelve-month wait.

What Andrew did not know when he chose not to tell his doctor that he had once been a heavy drinker was that his status as a nondrinker increased the likelihood that he would someday develop liver cancer. What happens with a former alcoholic is that once he stops drinking, his liver tries to heal itself by generating new tissue, something it did not attempt while the person was still drinking. There is something about the regeneration process that encourages cancer-producing changes in the genetic structure of the cells, and it generally takes about ten years for those mutated cells to be recognized as cancer.

Would Andrew have been better off if he had continued drinking? No—statistically, patients with alcoholic cirrhosis who die of liver cancer are about ten years older than patients who die of noncancer causes. If Andrew had continued to drink past the age of sixty, it is likely that he would have died of complications of cirrhosis well before he turned seventy.

Andrew's case underlines the difficult choices associated with being a senior with cirrhosis. He stopped drinking and that bought him more time, but more time in his case meant an increased likelihood that he would develop liver cancer. Andrew didn't exactly choose the latter option, but that was the one that life gave him.

What seniors need to know about cirrhosis

One age-based study on patients with hepatitis C found significant differences between patients sixty-five and older and those sixty-four and younger. The older patients were less likely to undergo a biopsy and less likely to receive treatment. Nearly 45 percent of the younger patients refused treatment or did not return for a second appointment, compared to 32.5 percent of the older patients, but among those who did return for treatment, nearly 34 percent of the younger patients received treatment, compared to less than 10 percent of the older patients.

What that study says to me is that the older patients were more conscientious about their health and displayed more cooperation with their doctors than the younger patients, but when it came to treatment, they were considered less desirable by their doctors than their younger counterparts. There are probably several reasons for that. That same study indicates that 41 percent of the younger patients who agreed to therapy received a sustained response, while only 25 percent of the older group experienced a sustained response. Doctors asked nearly 36 percent of their younger patients to undergo biopsies, compared to only 14 percent of their senior patients.

As with younger patients, the prognosis depends on the cause of the cirrhosis. Your survival time will be longer if your cirrhosis was caused by one of the autoimmune disorders such as autoimmune hepatitis or primary biliary cirrhosis than if it was caused by hepatitis B or C, or by alcohol consumption. However, among patients with autoimmune disorder, the survival rate is higher for those under sixty-five than for those over sixty-five.

After pondering the dreadful things that can happen to you as a result of cirrhosis, it is helpful to remember that your age will not disqualify you for a transplant—and if you do undergo a transplant, your survival rate will be comparable to that of younger patients. You may have to strongly advocate for yourself to get to the point where you can receive a transplant, but once you reach that point, you will be on equal footing with the twenty-five- or thirty-five-year-old who may have had an easier journey.

Other factors that affect senior patients:

○ Salt-restricted diets are less desirable for seniors since it makes food less tasty and may stifle the appetite.

○ Low-protein diets in older patients, especially if they are showing signs of encephalopathy, should be avoided since such patients are probably already undernourished to begin with.

○ Older patients do not tolerate beta-blockers as well as younger patients and may require different treatment for the prevention of bleeding varices.

○ Encephalopathy can be easily confused with senile dementia in senior patients.

○ Diuretics have to be adjusted more carefully because they pose greater risks of electrolyte disturbances in seniors.

○ Cirrhosis-related infections are easier to miss in seniors and more difficult to treat once diagnosed.

Things seniors can do to improve their odds

Be frank with your doctor. Doctors are only human. They know from experience that younger patients usually respond better to therapy and that makes them a better investment. Throughout their education as doctors, medical students are repeatedly reminded that one of their greatest responsibilities is to do no harm to their patients. That is a major concern for doctors with senior patients.

If you are sixty-five or older, your doctor is going to be reluctant to put you through the same aggressive treatment plan that she uses with younger patients. Your job is to let her know that you are willing to accept the increased risks that accompany some procedures and treatments, if, indeed, that is the way you feel.

When my grandfather was in his eighties, he went to see a doctor because of severe hip pain. After an examination, he was referred to a surgeon for a hip replacement. At first the surgeon was reluctant to proceed, citing my grandfather's age. The surgeon asked, "How long do you want to live?"

"Longer than this," answered my grandfather.

The surgeon performed the surgery (my grandfather was the oldest person he had ever operated on for this particular procedure) and my grandfather lived another twelve years, proving the worth of the surgery.

Seniors newly diagnosed with cirrhosis should have a frank discussion with their doctor about their attitudes toward treatment. Your doctor probably won't tell you outright if he or she is opposed to certain treatments for seniors, but you can gain insight into their thinking by asking two direct questions:

Am I too old for a transplant?

Am I a candidate for surgery if I experience bleeding in my esophagus or stomach?

If your doctor's answer to the first question is yes and to the second question is no, you might want to get a second opinion.

Avoid isolating yourself. Today, living longer can mean living alone longer, which can put seniors at increased risk for depression, destructive behavior, and suicide. The most insidious aspect of senior isolation is that it typically occurs through attrition, which means that it is seldom planned. Seniors measure passing time by the number of friends and relatives they lose each year. Many seniors find themselves in the position of having outlived all of their friends and family members.

Seniors face isolation in a variety of ways. Some turn to alcohol or antidepressants (50 percent of all sedatives prescribed in the United States are used by seniors). Some turn to gambling, which initially gives them a thrill because they are surrounded by people—but later that thrill can change to addiction as they find themselves unable to say no. Others regress to the emotions familiar to them from earlier in life and engage in a variety of risky behaviors, ranging from bad financial investments to self-destructive relationships with the opposite sex.

In many ways, isolation will be as great a threat to your survival as your cirrhosis. It is important that you do what you can to decrease your isolation. Spend more time with family members, even if it means inviting yourself into their homes. Make new friends. Those elderly bird-watchers that hike past your home in their silly outfits could be a lifesaver for you, so instead of laughing at them, grab your camera, even if it's out of film, and race outside to join them. I've never met a bird-watcher who didn't welcome strangers.

Since the negative effects of isolation—depression and an accompanying lowered resistance to infection due to a compromised immune system—will decrease your odds of fighting off serious complications, if they develop, it is essential that you do everything you can to avoid putting yourself in that position.

Isolation is not your friend, so do not allow it to become a part of your life.

IN A SENTENCE:

If you are a senior with cirrhosis, let your doctor know how aggressive you want her to be with your treatment.

learning

Dealing with Your Employer

Once I got over the trauma of my diagnosis,
the question I kept asking myself was
'What do I tell my boss?'

—MAGGIE W.

IF YOU work for a company with fifteen or more employees, or if you work for any federal, state, or local agency, you may be protected against discrimination under the Americans with Disabilities Act (ADA). The ADA applies to individuals who have impairments that "substantially" limit major life activities such as seeing, speaking, hearing, walking, breathing, performing manual tasks, learning, and caring for oneself.

The ADA prohibits discrimination in all employment practices, including job application procedures, hiring, firing, promotions, compensation, and training. The act provides equal-opportunity protections to individuals with disabilities similar to those provided to individuals on the basis of race, color, sex, national origin, age, and religion.

There are some diseases that the U.S. Department of Justice, which is responsible for enforcing the ADA, along with the Equal Employment Opportunity Commission, have identified as falling under federal guidelines. These include epilepsy, paralysis, HIV infection, AIDS, hearing or visual impairments, mental retardation, and some learning disabilities. Also included are mental illness, cancer, and "limiting impairments" such as a severe facial disfigurement.

Not included under the guidelines is cirrhosis. There have been instances in which individuals with cirrhosis have received protection under the act, but those cases involved people whose cirrhosis was caused by an active hepatitis virus. With no federal guidelines in place regarding cirrhosis, it has fallen to the courts to interpret the law.

In a 2000 ruling, the U.S. Seventh Court of Appeals found that cirrhosis caused by chronic hepatitis B was not a disability. Further, the court determined that liver function was not a major life activity, but rather a characteristic of the impairment. Of course, there will not be a definitive ruling on whether cirrhosis is a covered disease until the U.S. Supreme Court takes on the matter.

As of this writing, it would appear that if you have cirrhosis, your best chance of receiving ADA protection against discrimination will be if your cirrhosis was caused by hepatitis C and is still active in your system, requiring regular treatment by a physician.

What are my rights with small companies?

The ADA does not offer protection to individuals who work for employers with fewer than fifteen employees. If that is your situation, your approach to your employment situation will be different than it would be if you worked for a government agency or a large company. Essentially, you will be *asking* for fairness instead of *demanding* it.

However, even in small companies, there are still legal protections in place for you since many states have laws that are even more favorable to employees than the federal law. In some states, similar protections are offered to employees who work for employers who have as few as four workers.

Since there are fifty different sets of laws concerning small employers (one for each state), you would need to research the laws in your state to know if you are protected. If your employment is terminated because of your diagnosis, you should talk to someone in the state attorney general's office to determine if any state laws have been violated and you should talk to an attorney to receive an opinion on whether you have grounds for a civil lawsuit against your employer.

Medical records protections

The Health Insurance Portability and Accountability Act of 1996 (HIPAA) prohibits health-care providers from giving information to your employer about your medical records. However, if an employer receives information about your medical records from another source, the employer is not obliged to protect the information under HIPAA's privacy guidelines.

The instances in which your employer can obtain medical information about you without your permission include:

○ Information related to pre- and post-employment drug testing
○ Information obtained as part of a workers' compensation program
○ Information obtained from a credit bureau check, whether the information is explicit or implied

Several federal agencies—the Federal Aviation Administration, the Department of Transportation, and the Federal Highway Administration—require doctors and others to disclose medical information to them about their employees. Such disclosures become part of the employee's employment file and are not protected by HIPAA's privacy guidelines.

What are medical records?

Anytime you see a doctor or undergo a medical test, information is generated that goes into your medical record. Included are your symptoms, your doctor's observations, lists of your medications and the prescribed dosages, and the treatments prescribed for you. *Everything* you say or do while in a doctor's office or hospital testing facility is subject to inclusion in your medical records.

Some doctors are compulsive note takers. By that I mean they dictate or write down your exact words, even if the conversation had nothing to do with the medical problem. For example, if you confide to your doctor during a moment of stress that you are guilty of a marital infidelity or that you suspect your partner of being guilty of a marital infidelity, the chances are pretty good that the doctor will include that conversation in his notes about your office visit.

If you were treated for a venereal disease while you were in college and you tell your current doctor about it ten, twenty, or thirty years later, that experience will become part of your medical record, even if the doctor who originally treated you did not include that information in his or her notes.

What should I tell my employer?

There is no "one size fits all" answer to that question. As we have already seen, you have few guaranteed rights as a cirrhosis patient and the rights you do have vary from state to state. The knee-jerk answer is, "Tell your employers nothing—it's none of their business!" The more thoughtful answer would be, "Tell your employer anything that might be of help to you."

If you have a history of disputes with your employer, you obviously will want to be careful about what information you provide about your disease, or even whether you disclose that you have a chronic disease. Your employer does not have a right to know. However, if you have a good relationship with your employer, one that is marked by mutual respect, you might want to be upfront about your condition so that your employer does not hear about it from a third party. In that type of controlled situation, you will be able to explain that your long-term prognosis is good and you do not expect your disease to affect your work performance in any way.

How to protect your privacy rights

○ Be careful what you sign while in your doctor's office. The consent and disclosure forms they ask you to sign are for their protection, not yours.

○ Never discuss your disease in e-mails sent from work, since your employer has the right to monitor those messages.

○ Be careful what you say about your disease while talking on cordless or cell phones, since you never know who might be listening in.

○ Be discreet when you are exchanging comments with others in Internet chat rooms. Don't write anything that you would not want your employer to read.

IN A SENTENCE:

> *Know your rights: employment decisions can affect the course of your treatment.*

living

The Healing Power of Love and Prayer

I KNOW doctors who swear by the power of love and prayer, and I know doctors who swear if you mention the power of love and prayer. Which doctors are right? Technically, both are right, since different scientific studies have proved that both sides of the debate are right, a revelation that probably says more about the unreliability of science than it does about the durability of love or prayer.

I refer to love and prayer in one breath, as if they were the same thing, but they are not, of course. The power that derives from love has its source in other people, and even animals, while the power that derives from prayer has as its source a personal faith in the willingness of a higher power to intervene in human events.

My experiences as a journalist did not make me a believer in healing through spiritual support, but my second career as a social worker did open my eyes to those possibilities. As a social worker I saw my share of depraved souls, to be sure, but I also saw the good things that could happen to children when they were removed from a negative environment and transplanted to a loving home. Love and prayer can heal the deepest of wounds, if given a chance.

After I received my first diagnosis—a misdiagnosis that had me dying of an assortment of cancers—word of my illness spread in my hometown. I received word that members of the church that I had attended as a child were praying for my recovery. Soon cards started arriving on a regular basis, each card signed by those who had prayed for me. I had not seen some of the people who signed the cards for twenty-five or thirty years. Those cards and good thoughts provided me with a positive spiritual energy I had not experienced in many years. The thought of those people gathering in a church to utter my name was a powerful reminder to me that there are forces in life that we may never fully understand—forces that have the power to heal.

Of course, over the coming months, my diagnosis changed and my prognosis became much brighter. You may say that happened because I found two wonderfully talented doctors, but I also think that it was not an accident that I found those doctors. I think it took a great deal of love for people who had not seen me for many years to pray for my recovery—and I think that the combination of the two, love and prayer, took the "accident" out of the good things that subsequently happened to me.

Love as a healing power

> *Love in its essence*
> *is spiritual fire.*
>
> —EMANUEL SWEDENBORG

For centuries, poets have repaired broken hearts with well-chosen words of love, and there is a reason that our culture holds fast to the belief that, as the French song proclaims, "Love makes the world go 'round." As a culture we never needed further confirmation, but now, science has backed up our belief in the healing power of love. Consider the following examples:

In the 1980s, two Harvard psychologists, David McClelland and Carol Kirshnit, discovered that research subjects who viewed movies in which love was the theme experienced increases in levels of immunoglobulin-A in their saliva, chemicals that are the immune system's first line of defense against invading viruses.

Life insurance companies, our culture's commercial experts on longevity, learned many years ago that men who were kissed by their wives before they left for work are less likely to have an automobile accident on the way to work; they are also likely to live five years longer than men who do not receive good-bye kisses.

Dr. Bernie S. Siegel, a New England surgeon who wrote a best-seller entitled *Love, Medicine and Miracles*, believes that unconditional love is the most powerful stimulant of the immune system: "I feel that all disease is ultimately related to a lack of love, or to love that is only conditional, for the exhaustion and depression of the immune system thus created leads to physical vulnerability."

Of course, humans do not hold an exclusive trademark on unconditional love.

Show me a cirrhosis patient who has a pet—or daily access to someone else's pet—and I will show you a patient who is at an advantage in his recovery. An Australian study of six thousand patients at the Baker Medical Research Institute found that patients with pets had lower blood pressure and a lower cholesterol level than patients without pets, thus providing the pet owners with a reduced risk of heart disease. American studies, too, have found that coronary patients who own pets live longer than their pet-less counterparts. Other studies have found that pet owners:

- Live longer than people without pets
- Are less lonely than non–pet owners
- Have higher self-esteem

What should be of particular interest to cirrhosis patients is research that indicates that patients who have loving relationships with their pets are more likely to see positive changes in their immune system. As a liver patient, that should be of great interest to you.

Why are pets good for us?

I think it is because each of us has a need to touch other living organisms, and a need to give and receive unconditional love. There is probably a scientific basis for that, but who cares, really? We don't have to understand the molecular basis for the benefits that can be derived from pets. All we have to do is believe in them—and they will make themselves known to us.

Prayer as a healing power

God warms his hands
at man's heart when he prays.

—John Masefield

Scientific evidence regarding the healing power of prayer is mixed, depending on your definition of prayer. If you define prayer as something that someone else does on your behalf, or something that you do on the behalf of others, then you will find mixed scientific evidence in support of its effectiveness. However, if you define prayer as a personal communication with a higher power, undertaken for your personal benefit, you will find that scientific research is more supportive of your efforts.

The now-defunct U.S. Office of Technology Assessment (OTA) once undertook a survey of ten years' worth of issues of the *Journal of Family Practice* in an effort to reach a conclusion about prayer and religious beliefs. It found that 83 percent of the studies reported in the publication found a positive effect on physical health. In a second study, the OTA reviewed twelve years of issues from two psychiatric journals and tabulated the following breakdown on studies that measured the effects of religion on mental well-being: 92 percent show a benefit, 4 percent were neutral, and 4 percent showed harm.

A 1988 clinical trial conducted at a San Francisco hospital coronary care unit found that seriously ill patients who were prayed for were less likely to need antibiotics and suffered fewer complications than those who were not. However, a ten-year study that involved more than 1,800 patients and was published in the April 2006 issue of the *American Heart Journal* concluded that prayers offered by strangers had no effect on the recovery of people who were undergoing heart surgery. Dr. Charles Bethea, a coauthor of the study and a cardiologist at Integris Baptist Medical Center in Oklahoma City, said at a press conference called to explain the results, "One conclusion from this is that the role of awareness of prayer should be studied further."

Clearly, science cannot make up its mind whether there is a scientific explanation for the benefits of prayer. Is that surprising? Science cannot make up its mind if there is a scientific explanation for the creation of great literature, great art, or great music, the creative cornerstones of our society, so why should it be able to decipher the mysteries associated with prayer?

Meanwhile, there is plenty of anecdotal evidence that prayer is beneficial. Dr. Edward Hill, a former president of the American Medical Association, once told me about one of his patients who had inoperable lung cancer. It distressed him that there was nothing further he could do to help her, but when he explained that to her, he found her response surprising. She told him not to worry about it. She planned to spend her remaining days in prayer.

When the woman returned to his office a month later, she reported that all of her symptoms had gone away. Stunned, Dr. Hill ran a series of X-rays that disclosed that the tumors in her lungs had simply disappeared. The woman credited her miraculous recovery to the power of prayer. Dr. Hill was at a loss to explain it any other way.

I don't know whether the woman had a significant other she talked to about her disease, or whether she had family members with whom she shared her thoughts, but she clearly engaged in a conversation with God through prayer, and that communication proved to be therapeutic for her. There is no guarantee that prayer will cure your cirrhosis, but there is evidence that "talking to God" can counter the negative effects of isolation and provide you with the inner resources you will need to combat your disease.

Frankly, I don't think that science will ever make sense out of prayer. There are some things in life that must be accepted only on faith. Healing falls in that category.

In the Christian tradition, what made Jesus's ministry unique was his willingness to celebrate the healing attributes of love. For Jesus, disease was the enemy. It is the reason that he incorporated healing into the day-to-day activities of his ministry. "If the Good News is that Christ came to save all men, then the power to save has to be there," writes Father Francis MacNutt, author of *Healing*. "If the power to save man extends to the whole person, part of the very message of salvation is that Christ came to heal us—spirit, mind, emotions, and body."

Christians do not have a patent on healing. All of the world's major religions—Judaism, Islam, Buddhism—believe in the healing power of prayer. The Harvard Medical School sponsored a conference in 1996 called "Spirituality and Healing in Medicine." Among the speakers was Rachel Cowan, director of the Jewish Life Program, who said, "When we are sick, we rely on doctors for the best medical care available, but we also understand that healing takes place in the mind and soul, in the context of a caring community. . . . Jewish healing rituals and practices help us find the

inner strength to go on, to become active partners in improving the physical and mental condition of our lives. They help the ill person emerge from
the feeling of isolation and helplessness that illness imposes on so many."

The Islamic tradition of using prayer for healing is perhaps not as well
known in the West, but it is documented in the Koran, such as when a
companion of the Holy Prophet (Mohammed) complains of stomach pain,
to which the prophet advises him to "stand up and pray because healing is
in prayer."

Healing recommendations

One of the most important things you can do as a cirrhosis patient is to
develop a positive outlook about your recovery. Your doctor wants you to
take her advice on medical matters and she wants you to do what you can
to make your body receptive to the treatment that she prescribes. Two of
the most potent weapons you have at your disposal for creating a healing
environment within your body are love and prayer. With that in mind, I
offer the following suggestions:

- If you are religious, pray daily for your recovery. If you are not reli-
gious, do not discourage others from praying for you, whether they are
praying to Yahweh, Jesus, Allah, Buddha, or some other religious deity.
- Give love to those closest to you, and accept their love in return,
unconditionally.
- Mend fences with family members with whom you have become
estranged.
- If you do not have a pet, get one—and watch as it transforms your life.
- Avoid people with negative attitudes.
- Gravitate toward people with positive attitudes.
- Forgive those who have hurt you. Harboring suppressed anger is one
of the worst things you can do to your immune system.
- Seek out groups of people—support groups for cirrhosis patients,
religious discussion groups, community action groups dedicated to
public projects, etc.

IN A SENTENCE:

Love, prayer, and the support of others can be potent influences on your recovery.

Alternative Treatments

*I have taken every medication prescribed
by my doctor, but nothing seems to work.
My cirrhosis appears to be getting worse.
Should I try some of the herbal medicines?*

—LIZ G.

ALTERNATIVE THERAPY is any treatment that is not
within the bounds of traditional medical therapies. The popularity of alternative therapies in the United States has
increased dramatically in recent years, so much so that if you
added up all the visits that Americans make each year to alternative practitioners and added up all the visits they make to
medical doctors, the alternative practitioners would have the
more impressive numbers.

It is not surprising that institutional acceptance of alternative therapy has followed such widespread public acceptance.
The National Institutes of Health has conducted seminars on
alternative medicine. There has been increased public and private funding for research in alternative therapies. More and
more insurance companies are agreeing to cover the costs of
visits to alternative practitioners.

In 1993, the *New England Journal of Medicine* published the
results of a study conducted by Harvard University researcher

David Eisenberg, a medical doctor, who found that one in three American adults had used some form of unconventional medicine. The most frequently cited were techniques that fell in the mind/body category.

Subsequently, a study documenting trends from 1990 to 1997 was conducted by the Center for Alternative Medicine Research and Education at Beth Israel Deaconess Medical Center in Boston. This study found that the probability of users visiting an alternative medicine practitioner increased from the one in three cited in the Harvard study to 46 percent. Additionally, the study concluded that Americans made more visits to alternative medicine practitioners than to primary care physicians.

If you go to any large drugstore in the United States, you will find shelf after shelf of herbal remedies for every disease imaginable. Unfortunately, there is a line of thinking in the United States that considers anything sold in a drug or health food store as safe, since "they," meaning the government, would not allow anything harmful to be sold. That is a myth, of course. There is no government regulation of food supplements and herbal remedies. The government's position is "Buyer beware." Just because your local drugstore sells items that can be put into your mouth does not mean that you should do so—so be cautious.

This chapter will focus on alternative or natural remedies being used to treat liver diseases. Some of them have been used for hundreds of years. It's fine for cirrhosis patients to keep an open mind about such remedies, but also observe the medical doctor's dictum to "do no harm" in the process. Before you consume herbal products or submit to alternative procedures, you should research them carefully and you should always discuss your plans with your doctor.

However, as alternative therapy is not something that you should undertake without your doctor's knowledge, this may create a problem for you in another way. Although more and more doctors are accepting of an integrated approach to healing that includes herbs and food supplements, some remain adamantly opposed to any kind of alternative therapy. Your relationship with your doctor is similar to the relationship you have with your significant other in the sense that you don't want to be "unfaithful" to the relationship by doing things behind the other person's back. If your doctor is opposed to experimenting with alternative therapy for any reason, you will have to decide what is more important—the good relationship you have with your doctor or the possible benefits of alternative therapy. In that case, you may want to seek the opinion of another physician.

If you are considering adding alternative therapy to your treatment, the following are some topics that you should discuss with your doctor:

○ Mention specific herbs or treatments that you are considering and ask your doctor's opinion on their effectiveness and risks.

○ Ask if any of the therapies you are considering will interfere with the effectiveness of the medications you are already taking.

○ Ask your doctor if he or she thinks that your use of alternative therapies will affect, in any way, your insurance coverage for approved medical procedures.

Being a cirrhosis patient is all about making choices you never thought you would have to make. The problem with this disease is that most people who have it feel fine—right up until the moment they experience serious complications, such as bleeding varices or encephalopathy, which invariably lead to being placed on the transplant list. Alternative therapies offer hope to many and they should not be discounted without good reason. Neither should they be pursued without an awareness of the possible consequences. It's a fine line, but so is everything associated with cirrhosis.

Timing is an important factor in your decision to use alternative therapies. Do you want to experiment with them while you are in relatively good health and thus better able to withstand any "mistakes" in judgment—or do you want to wait until there is evidence that the standard medical therapies you have been using are losing their effectiveness?

In other words, do you see alternative therapy as a last resort or as a means to accelerate the progress that you are making with traditional medical therapy? If it is the former, you probably are not overly concerned about your doctor's opinion. If it is the latter, it would be prudent for you to be sensitive to your doctor's recommendations and follow that old frontier saying: "Dance with the one that brought you."

Menu of alternative therapies

Acupuncture. Acupuncture is the insertion of very small needles into the skin at sites called acupuncture points. Each point is a specific location on a network of meridians or channels. Ancient Chinese medical practice has it that there are fourteen major meridians in the body that connect the skin with important internal organs. People who are ill are thought to have energy blockages in the meridians that connect their organs. The needles are believed to cleanse those blockages by instigating a harmonious energy flow.

Acupuncture has been a part of mainstream medicine in Asian countries such as China and Japan for hundreds of years, but only recently has it come into widespread use in the United States. Today more than ten million acupuncture treatments are administered each year in the United States by thousands of licensed acupuncturists.

Does acupuncture work? There is no shortage of people willing to swear that it helped them with their cirrhosis, but thus far the scientific studies have been mixed, primarily because the nature of the treatment makes it difficult to use appropriate controls, such as placebos, to verify the procedure's effectiveness. However, the National Institutes of Health (NIH) has seen "promising results" in the use of acupuncture for postoperative and chemotherapy nausea and vomiting, and in postoperative dental pain. The agency lists other areas in which the procedure may be useful as an adjunct treatment or an acceptable alternative: addiction, stroke rehabilitation, headache, menstrual cramps, low back pain, carpal tunnel syndrome, and asthma.

The main area of interest for some cirrhosis patients is alcohol and drug addiction. In a 1997 report, the NIH recognized the effectiveness of acupuncture in encouraging patients to continue with their detox programs. Patients who underwent acupuncture, according to NIH, continued with the program longer than patients who did not. The report concluded: "This is very important since attendance is essential for the success of treatment."

Ozone therapy. Advocates of **ozone therapy** maintain that viruses of the type that cause hepatitis thrive in an environment that is low in oxygen. They reason that the best way to kill the viruses is to subject them to greater than normal amounts of oxygen. The vehicle they use to do that is ozone, which is made up of three oxygen molecules, as compared to the two oxygen molecules that are found in atmospheric oxygen.

Many doctors are opposed to this type of therapy, including Dr. Melissa Palmer, who writes, "If ozone can actually kill viral cells, it would also have the potential to kill healthy human cells. Therefore ozone therapy for people with hepatitis or other live diseases cannot be recommended at this time."

Metabolic therapies. These therapies are based on a belief that the cause of all diseases is the accumulation of harmful chemicals in the body. Specifics vary, but most therapies in this category are based on the ingestion of carrot juice and so-called cleansers such as coffee enemas. There is no evidence that any of these therapies are helpful to cirrhosis patients, but there is evidence that the increased levels of vitamin A found in carrot juice could be harmful. Likewise, coffee enemas could cause dehydration and result in constipation, a condition that could result in increased toxins in the bloodstream.

Popular herbs sometimes used by cirrhosis patients

Milk thistle (silymarin). This is by far the most widely used herb for liver disease. Derived from a plant that originated in Kashmir and then spread all over the world, it has been used for hundreds of years to treat disease. Herbalists claim that **milk thistle** is an effective treatment for liver disease because: (1) it protects the liver from free radicals, which damage liver cells, and (2) it promotes the production of new liver cells to replace the damaged ones.

Some studies have suggested that the herb is helpful for people with alcoholic cirrhosis and is successful in lowering liver enzyme levels in those patients, but other studies have indicated that the herb might cause liver-cell death. One study performed on animals indicated that milk thistle increased the production of ribonucleic acid, one of the building blocks needed for the production of new liver cells. To the best of my knowledge, there have been no experimental studies done with humans to confirm milk thistle's effect on the production of ribonucleic acid.

The most encouraging thing about milk thistle is that there are no reports of major side effects associated with the herb. Its curative powers seem to be strongest among people suffering from acute mushroom poisoning, alcoholic liver disease, or liver disease caused by the toxic effects of prescription drugs. It does not appear to be effective against viruses such as those that cause hepatitis B or C; it may lower enzyme levels in patients with those viruses, but it does not destroy the virus or eradicate it from the body.

If you take milk thistle, it may be helpful for you to know that the *Physicians' Desk Reference (PDR) for Herbal Medicine* recommends 200 to 400 mg of the herb daily. However, Christopher Hobbs, a noted herbalist and botanist, prescribes up to 1 gram of milk thistle extract a day for patients with high liver enzyme levels (150 or higher). He says: "I have never seen any appreciable side effects at this dosage, even when the herb is taken for extended periods." For more information about Hobbs's use of milk thistle and for information about herbs that he recommends to cool the liver and reduce inflammation, I suggest you refer to his book, *Natural Therapy for Your Liver*.

Licorice. This is not the candy, but rather the powerful root of the *glycyrrhiza glabra* plant, which is highly regarded as an effective treatment for various liver disorders. Some studies have shown that the herb stimulates production of the body's natural supply of interferon, one reason why the Japanese use it to treat hepatitis. When injected intravenously, it can apparently lower liver enzyme levels.

Despite the herb's popularity, it can cause a number of disturbing side effects, including high blood pressure, reduced potassium levels, and fluid retention. Perhaps for those reasons, the *PDR for Herbal Medicines* recommends that the herb not be used by people with chronic hepatitis, cirrhosis, or cholestatic liver disease. Autoimmune hepatitis patients who take prednisone should never use the herb, since it may interact with the drug in such a way as to elevate the effects of its dosage.

Licorice may be fine for liver patients whose disease has not progressed to cirrhosis, but its potential side effects mean that it should be avoided by cirrhosis patients who can ill afford problems with high blood pressure or fluid retention. If licorice is your herb of choice, you shouldn't take it without first consulting with your doctor.

Thymus extracts. This therapy is often considered herbal, even though thymus extract is made from the thymus glands of cattle and is sold as capsules and tablets. The reasoning is that since the thymus gland is involved in the regulation of the body's immune system, it can be formulated into a therapy for people with malfunctioning immune systems. Thymus extracts are promoted as a means to fight hepatitis C, but there is no clinical evidence to show that it works.

The most vocal supporter of thymus extracts is entertainer Naomi Judd, who has credited the therapy with helping her in her fight with hepatitis C. However, it should be noted that she has also taken interferon, followed a healthy diet, and used meditation and acupuncture as part of her treatment. For that reason, it is difficult to know how beneficial thymus extracts have really been to her. For more information about Judd's experiences with thymus extracts, I suggest you refer to her autobiography, *Love Can Build a Bridge*.

Kava. Let me be clear about this herb: if you have cirrhosis, kava can kill you. This is a plant indigenous to the islands in the South Pacific, where it is used to prepare a popular beverage. Supplements containing kava are promoted to relieve stress and tension, but the herb has made its way into the alternative-medicine cabinets of liver disease patients, perhaps because of the stress associated with the disease. In 2002, the U.S. Food and Drug Administration issued a consumer advisory about the herb in which the agency warned that it could cause severe liver injury, including cirrhosis. The advisory cited four patients who had required liver transplants after taking the herb.

Ginseng. This herb is usually sold in the form of capsules. Studies have indicated that ginseng can have some benefits for liver patients, but it has never been studied in association with hepatitis C, so its effect on that disease is unknown. Side effects include nosebleeds, nervousness, vomiting, and insomnia.

Green tea. The effective ingredient in green tea is catechin, a plant chemical that has antioxidant properties. Experiments with rats have proved catechin effective in stabilizing cell membranes, an important consideration for patients with liver disease, but similar studies with humans have been inconclusive. Side effects in humans include fever and allergic rash. If you are wondering: yes, the black tea that is sold in the United States also contains catechin, but only in low concentrations.

IN A SENTENCE:

If you decide to try alternative treatments or therapies, please discuss your plans with your doctor.

living

What You Need to Know about Sex

To be perfectly honest,
after learning that I had cirrhosis,
sex was the last thing on my mind.

—GUNTHER H.

ONE OF the first clues that a primary care physician may have that a male patient has cirrhosis is a request for Viagra—and one of the first clues that a primary care physician may have that a female patient has cirrhosis is a request for a referral to a plastic surgeon for a breast augmentation to correct shrunken breasts.

Such requests, spurred by loss of interest in sex and breast atrophy in women, typically outdistance the more obvious physical symptoms of cirrhosis by many months—or even years. The liver's connection to a person's sexuality is indirect but ever present. It can occur through the release of toxins into the bloodstream that make the patient lethargic and less responsive than usual to sexual stimulation. It can occur through circulatory changes that affect blood flow (the most visible indication of cirrhosis is palmar erythema, a reddening of the palms; just as the liver can redden the palms, it can affect blood flow to every part of the body, including the sexual organs). And it can occur through troublesome liver-related digestive problems that supersede sexual activity in importance to the patient.

When the minister performing the marriage ceremony urges the couple to stay together "in sickness and in health, to love and cherish, from this day forward until death do us part," it is with the realization that health issues can have a profound effect on a relationship. In the case of cirrhosis, the effect is often subtle, indirect, and difficult to identify. It is the vagueness of it all that is so harmful to a relationship. All an individual knows is that there is a change in his or her sexual relationship.

If loss of intimacy is the first casualty of liver disease, then self-blame is usually the first reaction to that loss. That's because the popular men's and women's magazines that promote solutions to sexual problems on the cover hardly ever refer to the disease-related causes of sexual dysfunction. As a result, an individual tends to play the blame game when the quality of his or her sex life changes. Sometimes they blame their partner. Sometimes they blame themselves.

Cirrhosis and men

> *My problem wasn't that I couldn't have sex.*
> *I could. There was no problem there.*
> *My problem was that I just didn't want to have sex.*
>
> —SAM B.

About 2 percent of the men in the early stages of liver disease experience impotence or erectile dysfunction, a percentage that is equal to the statistical incidence among healthy, middle-aged men without liver disease. Among the 2 percent who experience the problem it is a huge concern, but for the remaining 98 percent it is more of a potential threat that looms in their consciousness.

Of more concern to male cirrhosis patients is the loss of libido associated with the disease. There are many reasons why male cirrhosis patients may experience a loss of interest in sex. Some of the reasons may be physical in nature. Cirrhosis lowers testosterone levels in males while increasing estrogen levels. The physical manifestation of that can be seen in breast development. Other changes that take place, which often are a blend of physical and emotional factors, include testicle shrinkage; decreased muscle mass and redistribution of body fat in a manner that is consistent with female body shapes; and loss of body hair.

Other factors can add to the above-mentioned problems:

○ If the cirrhosis was caused by alcohol consumption, the dysfunction will be amplified by the alcohol use. Alcoholics typically experience sexual dysfunction even without cirrhosis, but if you add cirrhosis to that situation, the libido becomes almost unrecognizable.

○ Drug therapy: many drugs used in the treatment of cirrhosis, such as prednisone, have impotence as a side effect.

Cirrhosis and women

This may not make sense.
I found that I needed sex, but I didn't
want sex. How do you explain that to your partner?

—BARBARA H.

Women with cirrhosis apparently have normal sexual function unless their disease is caused by alcoholism or hepatitis C. Female alcoholics without liver disease often experience a decreased interest in sex, so it is not surprising that female alcoholics with cirrhosis also report a loss of interest in sex.

Breast atrophy in women appears to be a common early warning symptom of cirrhosis, but authorities differ on how prevalent it is (some studies say it is as high as 75 percent). Women who practice breast self-examination techniques frequently as a means to screen for cancer will notice breast atrophy earlier than women who do not practice self-examination, but since they are screening for lumps and growths, they may not be concerned by breasts that seem to be getting smaller.

Typically, a woman with atrophying breasts will attribute it to growing older or losing weight (if she is on a diet) or to normal hormonal changes. It will affect her sex life if she feels it makes her unattractive or if her partner comments on the changes in a negative way. Her solution may be to talk to her doctor about a breast augmentation. An alert doctor will want to determine the cause of the hormonal changes that made the breasts atrophy, and that could lead to a liver enzyme test and eventually to cirrhosis.

Hepatitis C is a factor in decreased interest in sex for women because of the side effects of the primary drugs used to treat the disease—interferon and ribavirin. Both drugs cause vaginal dryness, which can cause pain during intercourse. That discomfort may become even more severe if the patient develops atrophic vaginitis, a condition in postmenopausal women that is characterized by decreased estrogen production. Two additional issues affect women with hepatitis C. First, intimacy and sexual activity may be affected by concerns about viral transmission between partners. Second, doctors worry about the drugs' potential to cause birth defects. For that reason, women must practice two methods of contraception while on treatment and for six months afterwards. That, too, has an effect on sexual activity.

Women with autoimmune hepatitis who are being treated with prednisone may experience a loss of interest in sex, but the cause usually has a psychological foundation related to the side effects of the drug. Among the adverse effects of prednisone are:

○ Increased body hair
○ Weight gain
○ Thinning of scalp hair
○ Changes in the menstrual cycle
○ Increased sweating

Barbara H. (quoted above) is a good example. After being on prednisone for a couple of months, she still had a strong need for sex in her life, but the twenty pounds she gained, the strips of hair that fell from her scalp when she showered, the increased body hair, and a change in her menstrual cycle that made her "time of the month" unpredictable all caused her to be less interested in sex. It was a self-image problem, to be sure, but it had a very real impact on her sex life.

Relationship issues

It is difficult to separate sexual issues from relationships issues. Sex is an important ingredient in any relationship. Any change in the frequency or quality of intercourse will be perceived by one partner to be a reflection of the relationship. If the changes are noted before a diagnosis of cirrhosis is made, the partner who has not lost interest in sex may jump to the wrong conclusions about the relationship.

Of course, the complexity of the sexual issue in cirrhosis patients will depend on whether the individual is single or in an exclusive relationship. If the individual is single and is not in a relationship, the issue does not have great immediacy. It goes without saying that single cirrhosis patients should use caution in starting up new relationships since the potential for rejection is greater because of the sexual issue.

Single cirrhosis patients who are involved in relationships face the same challenges as married patients—namely, to be diligent in not allowing their cirrhosis to damage their relationship with a loved one. Communication is important. Once a diagnosis of cirrhosis is made, it is essential that the partners discuss the sexual issues associated with the disease. You should be prepared to say, over and over again, "Honey, this disease may affect our sex life—if it does, just know that I love you and we will find a way to get through it."

Solutions

If you are having problems of a sexual nature, whether it is impotence or a loss of interest in sex, it is important to determine the cause of your problem. It is a subject that should be discussed with your doctor. Once a cause has been established, action can be taken to remedy the situation—or at least explain the situation until it reverses of its own accord. In matters of sex, information sometimes has a curative effect.

If you are male and the problem is caused by the drugs being used to treat your disease, your doctor may be reluctant to prescribe yet another drug to counteract the effect of the first drug. Viagra has proven effective in treating erectile dysfunction in males, but its interactions with the drugs used to treat liver disease have not been studied. For impotence, your doctor may be more comfortable prescribing a noninvasive remedy such as a vacuum device and retention ring. The vacuum is a hand- or battery-operated air pump attached to a plastic cylinder. The penis is inserted into the cylinder and subjected to the vacuum, which causes blood to rush into the penis and form an erection. Once the erection occurs, a rubber ring is fastened around the base of the penis to block the outflow of blood. Erections created this way are known to last for twenty minutes or longer, and the device has proved effective in 90 percent of cases.

If your cirrhosis is not caused by hepatitis or one of the autoimmune disorders, you may not be on any medication, in which case your doctor may be more willing to prescribe Viagra or a similar drug for your sexual problems, provided you have no complications associated with your cirrhosis.

Your doctor's first priority is to save your life. You should never put your doctor in the position of having to decide whether to save your life or provide you with a meaningful sex life. For men and women, the best solution to sexual problems associated with cirrhosis is counseling.

Should you be having sex?

The answer to that depends on the cause of your cirrhosis. In most instances, the answer is yes. If you are otherwise in good health, go ahead and knock yourself out. The primary exception involves hepatitis B and C.

Hepatitis B is easily transmitted through vaginal, oral, and anal sex. If you have hepatitis B, you should notify potential partners that you are infected and, if they agree to have sex with you, you should use condoms. If you have cirrhosis but no immunity to hepatitis B, you should not under any circumstances have sex with someone known to have hepatitis B. Even if you do have immunity, you should question your motives.

Hepatitis C is not as easily transmitted through sex as hepatitis B. The U.S. Centers for Disease Control and Prevention recommend that sexually promiscuous individuals use condoms to prevent contracting or spreading the disease, but studies done on the transmission of the virus among individuals in long-term, monogamous relationships have found the risk of infection to be low.

Of course, definitions of sex vary from person to person, so you should be wary of any type of sexual behavior that involves biting or scratching or binding—anything that could put you in contact with the other person's blood.

If you have cirrhosis and push the envelope in your sexual activities, you may be asking for trouble. The prudent choice is to use protection when you have sex, have sex only with people you trust to tell the truth about any infections they might have, and to steer clear of any sexual activity that would expose you to your partner's blood.

IN A SENTENCE:

> *If you notice a sexual problem, don't pretend it doesn't exist—talk to your doctor.*

learning

Becoming a Partner in Your Care: Conversation with an Expert— Dr. Charles Hall, Gastroenterologist

> *The most common symptom of liver disease is nothing at all. The second most common symptom is just general weakness and fatigue, which we all have anyhow.*
>
> —DR. CHARLES HALL

THE SUCCESSFUL treatment of any disease, but especially cirrhosis, is based on the relationship between the patient and the doctor. As patients, we all know, or at least we think we know, what qualities we want in a doctor. We seldom stop to think what qualities doctors want in their patients.

With that in mind, I sat down with Dr. Hall to discuss that issue—and others.

What qualities do you see in patients who do well?

Probably the most important thing is that patients do not have alcohol-related cirrhosis. Alcohol is toxic to the entire body and people who have alcohol-related liver disease have alcohol-related disease all over their bodies and it keeps them from responding as well to treatment. Within the bounds of non-alcohol-related liver disease, like cirrhosis and hepatitis, the most important thing is a good, healthy lifestyle and a good attitude.

Do you think a positive attitude is important?

I can't give statistical evidence, but anecdotally, from my point of view, it makes a world of difference. There is no question in my mind.

If a patient believes you can't help them, it makes your job more difficult, doesn't it?

It makes my job more difficult if they don't believe I am going to be able to help them or if they just don't believe they are going to be helped. If they are depressed and upset about being ill, which everyone is, and they can't get over that, then they are going to have a hard time. If they have a positive attitude and feel they can get better, there is no end to the good that can come from that.

What can cirrhosis patients do to help themselves?

To become as well educated as they possibly can. The more people know about what is going on with them, the better they can help me. That helps them to understand what their treatment is so that they will be able to do the treatment adequately and it also helps them to not be afraid. People who have hepatitis and liver disease tend to be scared to death when they first find out they have it. The more they read and understand it, the less fear they have. Education is the number-one thing.

Most of the patients I have tend to be well educated and they are Internet savvy. You can find a lot of crazy, bad information on the Internet, as you know. The Internet has good and bad points, but if you are savvy about what to look for and don't look at the crazy stuff, you can learn so much. People with hepatitis and liver disease need to learn as much about it as they can. The people I treat with liver disease, within a few months they know as much about it as I do—and that's the truth.

Cirrhosis is a master of disguise, isn't it?
The liver has so many functions, and symptoms of liver disease are so non-specific. The most common symptom of liver disease is nothing at all. The second most common symptom is just general weakness and fatigue, which we all have anyhow. So who would know?

Are patients like myself who have autoimmune hepatitis more likely to get other autoimmune diseases?
Yes, for reasons that are unclear. We don't know what causes the immune system to turn on the body with people who have rheumatoid arthritis, who have thyroid disease, who have Addison's disease. It doesn't necessarily mean that patients with one will get another, but there is an increased risk, higher than the general population.

How do you feel about alternative treatments?
You are talking about herbal therapies and things like that. For the most part, those treatments have never been shown to be helpful. I can't recommend them. Most of them are harmless, though. As long as they are not harmful to people and as long as people don't ignore helpful treatments, I don't see any harm.

So it could be helpful if it gave them a positive attitude?
Yes, absolutely . . . as long as they don't let it be their only treatment. I don't want someone like you taking bay leaves and not taking your medication. If you told me you were supplementing with vitamins and amino acid, I would say I have no evidence that it will help you but I don't have any evidence, either, that it will harm you and there is a lot about liver disease we don't understand.

How do you feel about experimental treatments?
Experimental drug therapy should not be done outside a clinical setting in an academic center. Someone like Dr. Fredric Regenstein [at Tulane Medical Center] is often involved in experimental studies and I think that's fine.

If you had cirrhosis, what would concern you the most?
What would concern me the most would be the possibility of liver cancer, because liver cancer is a higher risk in people with cirrhosis. You have to

check that every six months by doing a sonogram and alpha protein level test. That would be my biggest fear. The second would be that it might or might not progress and I might require a liver transplant somewhere down the road. That would be frightening to me because it is a big deal. But it is becoming more and more routine. The biggest fear I would have, as a physician, would be the fear of not having control over it—because what happens is going to happen. I cannot influence it. I can only wait and see what happens. We, as physicians, don't like to be out of control.

Dr. Hall's comments demonstrate the necessity of forming a partnership with your doctor in the treatment of your cirrhosis. Working separately, neither patient nor doctor can be effective in treating cirrhosis. One reason for that is the sheer complexity of the disease. It assumes multiple identities as it generates symptoms that sometimes can seem unrelated—and, for that reason, it requires constant monitoring.

Working together, patient and doctor can increase the odds of a successful outcome. One of Dr. Hall's strengths as a doctor is his ability to motivate patients to play an active role in their treatment. He wants your feedback, as will any good doctor who understands the importance of the partnership.

IN A SENTENCE:

What your doctor needs most from you is a positive attitude.

Finding Information and Support on the Internet

> *My doctor suggested that I use*
> *the Internet to find out more about cirrhosis.*
> *I did—and it helped some—but the real value*
> *for me was in the new friends I met*
> *in the online support groups.*
>
> —DALE W.

AS A patient, you now have an advantage that most didn't just ten years ago—the ability to instantly access information and support via the Internet. In 1995, only 27 percent of American homes had personal computers. The number jumped to 50 percent in 1998, to 56 percent in 2000, and then to 66 percent in 2001. Today it is thought to be around 70 percent. That translates to around 200 million Americans who have home access to computers and the Internet.

For people with serious illnesses such as cirrhosis, the Internet can provide a vast amount of information about the disease, news about new treatments and therapies, and an electronic portal through which cirrhosis patients can get in touch with other people who have the disease. The value of the last benefit should not be underestimated.

Randy H. handled his cirrhosis diagnosis with relative ease. He didn't break down and cry. He didn't blame himself, or God, for his misfortune. His biggest concern was his friends, none of whom responded in an appropriate way.

That bothered Randy for a long time, so much so that he went online to meet new friends in cirrhosis chat rooms and support-group sites. He started out by reading the postings of other patients. He was amazed that they often expressed the same frustrations he felt and had the same questions he had about his treatment options.

After several weeks of reading the postings of three individuals with whom he seemed to have the most in common, he contacted each of them by e-mail and began three new friendships that gave him the sort of satisfaction he had not experienced since high school. It took a while for him to figure it out, but, once he did, he realized that his old friends did not so much abandon him as they felt excluded from his experiences. He bonded so easily with his new cyber friends because they shared the same experiences.

The Internet provides unlimited opportunities for personal growth and a better understanding of your disease, but not all Web sites are created equal. The Internet is like a wilderness trail. It can take you to exciting places that will enrich your life in countless ways, but it can be dangerous if you lose your way and wander into hostile territory.

Finding what you need

The Internet can provide you with information in an instant that it would take you hours to obtain in a traditional library. It can provide you with advisories about new treatments and therapies, and you can literally obtain that information as quickly as your doctor can, unless your doctor is involved in research and maintains an ongoing dialogue with others conducting research in the same field. And it can put you in touch with other cirrhosis patients around the world, people who have the same fears and concerns, and who may already have experienced complications that you have not.

If it is other people you want to reach on the Internet, the best way to proceed is simply to type the phrase "cirrhosis support group" into a search engine such as Google or Yahoo, and then wade through the responses until you come across one that interests you. You will be surprised at how easy it is to engage others in e-mail conversation. Most of them will be just like you—eager to talk to someone about their experiences. Support-group sites have provided the foundation for strong friendships (and romances) among cirrhosis patients, and you owe it to yourself to at least give it a try.

If it is information, not friendship, that you want, you must be selective in the sites you visit. Generally speaking, sites that end in .org or .edu or .gov are more dependable than .com sites. I recommend that you begin your search at sites operated by established institutions. Examples include:

- U.S. Department of Health and Human Services (www.hhs.gov)
- American Association for the Study of Liver Diseases (www.aasld.org)
- American Liver Foundation (www.liverfoundation.org)
- Centers for Disease Control and Prevention (www.cdc.gov)
- National Center for Health Statistics (www.cdc.gov/nchs/fastats/liverdis.htm)
- National Institutes of Health (www.nih.gov)
- National Institute of Diabetes and Digestive and Kidney Diseases (www.niddk.nih.gov)
- Canadian Liver Foundation (www.liver.ca)
- American Gastroenterological Association (www.gastro.org)
- American Cancer Society (www.cancer.org)
- American Family Physician (www.aafp.org)
- National Institute of Mental Health (www.nimh.nih.gov)
- Wilson's Disease Association (www.wilsonsdisease.org)
- Cincinnati Children's Hospital Medical Center (www.cincinnatichildrens.org)
- Mayo Clinic (www.mayoclinic.org)
- U.S. Food and Drug Administration/Center for Devices and Radiological Health (www.fda.gov/cdrh/)
- RadiologyInfo (www.radiologyinfo.org)
- Tulane Center for Abdominal Transplant (www.tulanetransplant.com)
- Liver Transplant Program and Center for Liver Disease/University of Southern California Department of Surgery (www.surgery.usc.edu)
- American Medical Association (www.ama-assn.org)
- American Holistic Medical Association (www.holisticmedicine.org)

- ○ Hepatitis B Foundation (www.hepb.org)
- ○ Hepatitis Foundation International (www.hepfi.org)
- ○ (www.hepcfoundation.org)
- ○ Other, more commercial sites that are helpful include:
- ○ MedicineNet (www.medicinenet.com)
- ○ Merck Manual of Diagnosis and Therapy (www.merck.com)
- ○ *The New York Times* (www.nytimes.com)
- ○ Medscape (www.medscape.com)
- ○ eMedicine (www.emedicine.com)
- ○ Postgraduate Medicine (www.postgradmed.com)
- ○ WebMD (www.webmd.com)

Ways to determine if a Web site is legitimate

- ○ Are there advertisements on the site that claim to cure or treat ailments discussed on the site? If so, be skeptical of the information offered.
- ○ Does the site let you know who is providing the information and their qualifications for doing so? If not, be skeptical.
- ○ Does the site provide information that runs counter to what your doctor has told you? If so, look for independent verification of the information from additional sites, and discuss it with your doctor at your next visit.
- ○ Search engines are supposed to gather the most visited sites for presentation to you, but in reality they often accept payments from vendors who want their sites to have improved visibility. Sites labeled as "sponsored" should be viewed as advertisements.
- ○ When you visit commercial sites you will pick up "cookies" on your hard drive that will lead the site back to your computer via e-mails that offer to sell you liver-disease products. Such solicitations should be viewed with great skepticism.
- ○ Be careful when you enter chat rooms set up for cirrhosis patients. Computer predators often patrol such sites looking for vulnerable individuals for sexual or financial exploitation. Chat all you like, but draw the line at giving out personal information such as a mailing address or a telephone number.

Being cautious

Internet addiction. No one questions the positive benefits of the Internet, but cyberspace exploration is not free of negative consequences. Too much time spent on the Internet can contribute to isolation by allowing people to retreat into emotional castles, where one can engage in imaginary careers and relationships with anonymity and without the burden of personal accountability. Not only can the Internet increase risky social behavior and stand in the way of individuals developing close human relationships, it can also be as addictive as cigarettes, alcohol, or gambling. Of course, most of us can use the Internet without disastrous consequences, but for some people, it can lead to addiction.

In 1999, at a meeting of the American Psychological Association, Dr. Kimberly S. Young presented the results of a survey of nearly two thousand Internet users. It showed that 6 percent of those surveyed met the criteria for addiction. You might have an Internet addiction problem if you answer yes to more than one of the following questions:

- ○ Have you ever risked a relationship, a job, or a career opportunity because of the Internet?
- ○ When you are offline, do you ever think about what you are going to do when you are again online?
- ○ Have you ever lied to family or friends about how much time you spend online?
- ○ Do you feel moody or depressed if you try to cut back on the time you spend online?
- ○ Have you noticed that you are spending more time on the Internet than you did last month or the month before that?

At first glance, a 6 percent addiction rate does not sound like a large number, but when you apply it to 200 million Internet users, you arrive at 12 million addicts, not an insignificant number of souls lost in cyberspace.

Paul Gallant, a counselor at a Tucson addiction center, says that people are lured by the appeal of creating new identities for themselves:

"Your life may be really boring in reality, but online you're a competitive superhero." In a medium where information is limitless, even innocent inquiries can become obsessive, he says: "Say you're a wine connoisseur, you find this great site and it's linked to another great site. Fine, you've learned a lot more about wine. Then all of a sudden you realize six hours have gone by. You're obsessed with getting more and more information."

If you decide to use the Internet as a tool in your recovery, you should make an effort to avoid its addictive effects by setting a limit on the time you spend online. So how much time is too much? The answer does not lie in hours, but rather in your behavior. If you neglect your family, your job, or your spouse because you cannot tear yourself away from the Internet, then you are clearly spending too much time online. If your family, a loved one, or your employer is complaining to you, then that is a good indication that you should monitor your online time more closely.

Misinformation. Aside from the isolation effect that the Internet can have on cirrhosis patients, there is the problem of misinformation. Just because something is published on the Internet does not make it true. Unlike the traditional media—newspapers, magazines, television, etc.—most Internet sites are not supervised by an experienced editor.

If someone with a Web site believes that drinking the stew from boiled tennis socks will cure cirrhosis, he can present that information in such a way that it will appear to be reputable. Some sites owned by companies that sell alternative treatment therapies have sites that present information about cirrhosis in a convincing way, so far as symptoms, complications, and prognosis are concerned, but then you reach a point in the data when they pitch their product as a treatment for the disease. At that point you have to wonder if they have "doctored" the data to make their product more attractive.

If you are seeking information about cirrhosis on the Internet, be sure to take the source of the information into consideration. If the information comes from a site that is associated with a legal entity, such as the Mayo Clinic or the American Medical Association, the information is backed up by an organization that has a physical address and can be held accountable in a court of law. However, if the information comes from a site that is cloaked in anonymity, with no physical address or publicly named editorial board or board of directors, then you have no way of holding the site accountable for misinformation.

IN A SENTENCE:

> *The Internet can be an excellent resource and support system, but be sure to exercise appropriate caution.*

learning

Improving Your Odds: Conversation with an Expert—Dr. Fredric Regenstein, Hepatologist

Why do you think cirrhosis has a lower public profile than heart disease or cancer?

Several reasons. One, because of the common misconception that you only get cirrhosis if you drink too much. There is a negative perception that liver disease is related to alcohol, and that's one of the common things that a patient says when they come in and they are told they have liver problems, or they are told they have hepatitis. The first thing out of their mouth is, "Well, I don't drink. I never drank." Or, "How can I have liver disease? I thought you only got liver disease by drinking."

Another thing is that the second-largest cause of liver disease is viral hepatitis. Many people get viral hepatitis, especially hepatitis C, from previous substance abuse. So people who have hepatitis C in many cases don't want to be recognized, or they don't want it known because of the stigma associated with hepatitis, plus there is the issue that a person who has hepatitis may be contagious and people don't necessarily want that information disseminated—just like someone with HIV may feel they don't want people to know they have the disease because it might change the way people relate to them.

What do people not know about cirrhosis that would surprise them?
One common misconception is that once you have cirrhosis you are going to die imminently. That's not always the case. Another misconception is that if you have cirrhosis you should automatically feel bad. Some of the people who have cirrhosis don't know they have cirrhosis and they come in and say, "I don't feel that bad. Why am I not sicker?"

The biggest thing about this disease is its spectrum. It can extend from people who are completely asymptomatic, appear healthy, and have no major manifestations, to the other end of the spectrum, with people who are bedridden in the hospital, can't get out of bed, and literally have days to live. The other thing is that people sometimes mistake cirrhosis and cancer, and clearly they are not the same. Cirrhosis may predispose to cancer, but, in and of itself, it is not cancer.

Another misconception is over liver function. People want to know how much liver function they have left. They are told they have 20 percent of their liver function, or 15 percent of their liver function, and people don't understand that cirrhosis is a uniform process that pretty much involves the entire liver. You don't usually just get cirrhosis in one spot. Cirrhosis can't be removed or cut out. It is a process that involves the entire liver. The cirrhotic process itself is separate from liver function. You can have cirrhosis *and* a normally functioning liver, although the liver is anatomically scarred and damaged. For all intents and purposes it is functioning well, so there is a disconnect in that cirrhosis leads to problems or complications that are independent of function.

The complications it can cause are due to the fact that cirrhosis causes abnormalities in the way that blood flows through the liver, which is separate and distinct from the complications you get when the liver is not functioning. Most manifestations of cirrhosis really have to do with the fact that blood is not able to flow through the liver normally because of the structural changes that take place in the liver. The major complications that people run into—encephalopathy, fluid retention, varices—are related not to liver function, but to the fact that there is a detour and blood is bypassing the liver in many cases. That's something that people have a difficult time grasping.

What are your thoughts about alternative medications such as herbs and acupuncture?

I think herbs, or some herbal therapies, may be beneficial for liver disease, but there has not been a convincing scientific study to show that they are beneficial. I think they may be detrimental in situations where herbal therapies are substituted for proven therapies.

If you have a treatment for hepatitis and you forgo a treatment that can cure the hepatitis and take herbs instead, then I think you are doing yourself a major disservice. If, on the other hand, you failed treatment or you are not a candidate for treatment and you want to try herbal therapy, then I think it is perfectly reasonable if you have realistic expectations and you don't take a large number of herbs that are not pure or herbs of which you really don't know the effects.

The herb most commonly taken by patients with liver disease is milk thistle. Somewhere in the range of 40 to 60 percent of the people in the United States who have hepatitis or cirrhosis take milk thistle. The good news about milk thistle is that it is safe. The bad news is that it's really not clear if it's doing anything. Again, if you don't mistakenly forgo proven treatment to take an unproven treatment, then I think you are okay taking something like that. If you expect that to take the place of treatment, then you are being sort of foolish.

How big a problem is obesity when it comes to cirrhosis?

It's a big problem because the liver disease related to fatty liver is increasing. Fatty liver is associated with obesity, diabetes, insulin resistance, and the metabolic syndrome. The prevalence of these disorders in the United States population is on the increase, whereas the incidence of hepatitis B and C is on the decline.

What's the best thing that a patient can do to prepare themselves for a transplant?

Patients need to try to take control of their lives. They need to follow the directions of their physician. If the physician tells them they need to lose weight, that they need to control their diabetes, that they need to watch their salt intake, that they need to take their medications as prescribed, they need to follow those instructions. The key thing is finding a competent physician and basically doing everything that physician recommends.

If you start freelancing and doing things on your own, you are basically taking your life in your own hands.

What can a transplant patient do to improve their odds of a successful transplant?

They need to take care of themselves. Quit smoking. Stop drinking. Follow dietary recommendations. Take their medications. Adhere to the schedule for follow-up care.

At what point after a transplant can a patient feel they are out of danger of serious complications?

They are always at risk for complications because their immune system will always be suppressed. So they may be predisposed to more severe illnesses, infections, and other complications of the antirejection medications, and if they stop taking the antirejection medications because they feel that everything is okay, then they run the risk of rejection. It is a lifelong problem they are always at risk for, but in most cases it is manageable. It is certainly a worthwhile trade-off.

If you had cirrhosis, what would be your greatest concern?

It depends on what complications I had. The complications can be different in different people. For example, if you have cirrhosis and have large esophageal varices, the biggest concern will be bleeding from the esophageal varices. If you have cirrhosis and problems with fluid retention, and you are retaining fluid in your abdomen, the biggest danger in that situation may be an infection of the fluid.

Overall, the biggest threat to most cirrhotic patients is sudden, unpredictable death caused by a superimposed infection, which could be something, like pneumonia or appendicitis or a gall bladder attack, that requires emergency surgery and can cause the patient to spiral downward. Another threat would be an episode of bleeding from varices, which has a high mortality rate. And the third thing would be the unexpected development of cancer.

If you look at the complications, many of them could be predicted, because as a liver deteriorates, the doctor can see the deterioration in the lab work. The doctor can jump in and say, "Okay, you've reached the point where a transplant is on the horizon and we need to go ahead and do all the necessary tests to get you on the waiting list. The things that can happen suddenly and unpredictably don't follow a graduated progression—the sudden onset of a liver cancer, the sudden onset of bleeding. You could be functioning normally and have an episode of bleeding and die.

Under what circumstances would you recommend that a patient enroll in an experimental drug program?
I think there are advantages and disadvantages to experimental drug programs. If a person has no proven treatment alternatives, has ready access to an experimental treatment program, and is willing to try something which may or may not help, then they should participate. It is important for people to understand the potential risks and potential benefits. They should never feel pressured to participate. For patients with a disease where standard treatments are available, they must thoroughly consider the alternative therapies before agreeing to participate in an experimental drug program.

Do you see any experimental treatments on the horizon that show promise?
For generic cirrhosis, there is a class of drugs known as antifibrotics, which people have been looking at for many years. Progress is being made in that area, but I don't anticipate a breakthrough within the next three to five years. Down the road, I think that antifibrotics may ultimately be useful for patients with all types of cirrhosis.

There have been dramatic breakthroughs with hepatitis. If you go back to 1990, when the first drug for hepatitis C, interferon, was approved, the success rate was 5 percent. Now the success rate is almost 50 percent for eradicating hepatitis C and in improving cirrhosis, or reversing cirrhosis in some cases. As we get better treatments for hepatitis B and C, the success rate for treating people with cirrhosis will continue to improve; but for other forms of cirrhosis, the key breakthroughs are going to be in figuring out what the cause is and treating or controlling it—and, for the scar tissue, the treatment will be the antifibrotic agents.

IN A SENTENCE:

Patients can take control of their cirrhosis.

MONTH 11

When Treatment Fails: Finding a Transplant Center

ACTOR LARRY Hagman, star of the popular television series *Dallas* and *I Dream of Jeannie*, was sixty years old when he was diagnosed with cirrhosis in 1992, the result of thirty years of alcohol abuse. Three years later, a cancerous tumor was found on his liver, and he was placed on a transplant list at Cedars-Sinai Medical Center in Los Angeles.

There are two dates that Hagman says he will never forget: March 21, 1980, the day 350 million Dallas fans in over fifty countries tuned in to see who shot Hagman's character, J. R. Ewing—and August 23, 1995, the day he got a second chance for life with a liver transplant. The surgery was successful and he went for nine years with no reported problems. Then, in 2004, he learned that his new liver was diseased.

Hagman was honest about the reasons why. He had started drinking again, though he claimed that he was only having one pint of beer a month, "not for the buzz, but for the taste." His doctors recommended that he undergo surgery to cut away the diseased portion of his new liver but they cautioned him that the success rate for such surgical procedures was not high. At the time, Hagman referred to the problem as a "recurring infection," but his descriptions of the surgery are more consistent with a tumor removal. Hagman gave them the go-ahead.

Before the surgery, he telephoned each of his five granddaughters and chatted with them about their lives and how they were doing at school. "I love you," he said to each granddaughter and then signed off without telling them that he was about to undergo major surgery. "It was my choice to go ahead with the operation," he later explained to reporters. "But the choice was between that or dying . . . so I just made out a really good will." Hagman not only survived the surgery, he beat the odds. Two years later, in mid-2006, he was still going strong.

In 1995, the same year that Hagman received his transplant, baseball legend Mickey Mantle learned that he needed a new liver, the result of years of alcohol abuse and an active case of hepatitis. Two days after being put on the transplant list, he was given a liver transplant at Baylor University Medical Center in Dallas. Unfortunately, when doctors operated they learned that Mantle had a cancerous growth in his liver that had escaped detection by the various tests and scans he'd undergone.

Mantle died a few days after his surgery, ensued by a public uproar because he'd received a new liver so quickly. There were charges of favoritism, with many people wondering why the liver had not gone to someone with a better chance of survival. Others defended the surgery, including the *Houston Chronicle*, which published an editorial that brashly noted: "If the fact that he is Mickey Mantle had something to do with it, that is fine. . . . He is, after all, an American legend."

As a result of public concern about the fairness of the liver allocation system, it was changed in the late 1990s to provide a more equitable method of determining who gets available livers—and it has been updated several times since then.

When is it time to think about a transplant?

A liver transplant is not the sort of thing you think about at the last minute. The appropriate time to start thinking about it is as soon as you have your wits about you after you are told that you have cirrhosis—not that you will need a transplant soon, if ever.

The best time to bring up the subject with your doctor is when he or she has made a definitive determination of the cause of your cirrhosis. Be straightforward: "If it ever looks like I will need a liver transplant, where would you recommend that it be done?"

Your doctor may dance around that question for a moment or two, long enough to make positive comments about your prognosis, but once that is done, he or she will tell you the name of the transplant center to which they refer their patients. At that point, you might want to ask why they prefer that particular center.

Once you get home, you can investigate the center on the Internet and decide if it is where you would like to have transplant surgery, if it is ever needed. It would be prudent to investigate other transplant centers as well.

Cirrhosis is an unpredictable disease. It may be two years, five years, ten years before you need a transplant—or you may live into old age and die of something else. Meanwhile, you will feel better about the transplant procedure if you do your homework in advance.

How the current liver allocation system works

The United Network for Organ Sharing (UNOS) is the agency that oversees and coordinates liver transplants in the United States. It has a staff of three organ-placement specialists that operates in two twelve-hour shifts, with one specialist on call. When organs are donated, the procuring organization contacts UNOS directly, or it accesses the national transplant computer system, called UNet, through the Internet, so that information about the donor can be entered into the computer and matched with the recipients on the waiting list.

Once that happens, the potential matches are ranked according to medical criteria:

- O Blood type
- O Tissue type
- O Organ size
- O Medical urgency of the patient
- O Patient's time on the waiting list
- O Distance between the donor and the recipient

Based on the above criteria, an official at UNOS will contact the transplant center of the highest-ranked patient and offer the organ. If the organ is rejected by the transplant center, UNOS will move on to the second name on the list, and so on. Once the organ is accepted, transportation arrangements are made and the surgery is scheduled.

How do you get on the national waiting list?

As you would expect, your journey to the national waiting list begins with a referral from your doctor. The first step is for your doctor to contact a transplant center. She probably has a specific transplant center in mind that she will recommend to you. Several factors will enter into your doctor's choice:

- ○ Familiarity—your doctor will naturally want to refer you to the center with which she has the most experience.
- ○ Location—since evaluations, surgery, and postsurgery examinations will require many visits to the transplant center, your doctor will take travel time into consideration.
- ○ Expertise—not all transplant centers are created equal, since surgical success rates vary considerably from center to center.
- ○ Finances—some centers are more willing than others to work with patients who have inadequate insurance or no insurance at all.

If you do not like your doctor's choice of transplant center, you should discuss that with her and let her know if some of the criteria for choosing a center are more important to you than others. For example, if your doctor chooses a center that is five hundred miles away because of her relationship with the doctors, but you prefer a center that is only one hundred miles away, you should discuss it with her. Your doctor will not insist that you go to a particular center. She will make whatever arrangements you choose. Once you are evaluated by the transplant team at the center and found to be acceptable for their program, your name will be added to the waiting list.

Finding the right transplant center

There are more than two hundred transplant centers in the United States. Some are associated with university hospitals; some are associated with private hospitals. You can see a complete list at www.ustransplant.org; just look for the annual report on liver transplants done each year in the United States. The Web site offers a state-by-state list, complete with the number of transplants done yearly at each center.

It is permissible to be listed at more than one transplant center, but that does not improve your odds of receiving a donor liver any faster. The "matching" procedure goes at its own pace, regardless of how many centers have listed you as a patient.

Generally speaking, the more transplants a center does per year, the higher the experience level. Common sense tells you that you are better off with a surgeon who spends each day performing a specific surgery than with a surgeon who performs the surgery only on a monthly basis. As you might expect, the states that report the most liver transplants are California (more than seven hundred a year), with the University of California at Los Angeles Medical Center performing almost two hundred surgeries a year; New York (with more than five hundred), Pennsylvania (with more than five hundred), Florida (with more than five hundred), and Texas (with more than five hundred).

States that fall within the next tier (about two hundred transplants each year) include: Louisiana (with Ochsner Foundation Hospital and Tulane University Medical Center performing most of the surgeries), Michigan (with University of Michigan Medical Center performing most of the surgeries), and Ohio (with University of Cincinnati Medical Center performing most of the surgeries).

The American transplant surgeon with the highest visibility is probably Dr. Ronald Busuttil, who founded the transplant program more than twenty years ago at UCLA. Dr. Busuttil, who did his surgery residency training at Tulane, attracted a lot of attention in 2006 when it was disclosed that his income was $1.6 million a year, higher than the university's basketball coach. I, for one, find that gratifying. Of the 4,000 transplants that have been done at the center, Busuttil has performed nearly 3,000, which translates to an average of 136 surgeries a year. I mention Busuttil because it would be difficult to find a more experienced liver transplant surgeon in the United States. The vast majority of transplant surgeons have performed considerably fewer than 3,000 surgeries.

A 1998 analysis of survival rates at U.S. liver transplant centers found that the centers with the lowest survival rates were those that performed twenty-five or fewer transplants each year. The analysis, which was published by the Department of Health and Human Services at the request of UNOS, made it clear that there is a strong relationship between a center's success rate and the number of transplants it performs.

With that in mind, most experts concede that your odds are best at centers that perform twenty-five or more surgeries a year. However, there is no evidence that a center that performs one hundred surgeries per year is any better than one that performs forty or fifty surgeries per year, so you would not want numbers alone to be your reason for choosing a center. Other factors, such as location, postoperative care, and staff reputations are equally important and should be taken into consideration.

All of the major transplant centers have Web sites that will answer all of your questions. I strongly suggest that you explore the Web sites of the centers that seem the most attractive to you. Where you have a transplant is a decision that is entirely under your control. Try to make an informed decision.

IN A SENTENCE:

It's not too early to be thinking about a transplant center.

learning

If You Have to Have a Transplant

> *Just the thought of getting a liver transplant*
> *made me tense, but when the time came*
> *to have the surgery, everything was planned out*
> *so well that all I had to do was keep a positive attitude*
> *and climb aboard for the ride.*
>
> —WILLIAM T.

THINK OF your liver as the repository for a red-hot coal, which is the inflammation that threatens to shut down your system. It makes the inside of your liver red and tender, the same way that an inflammation on your arm or leg makes your skin red and tender.

Your doctor has spent the last year treating your inflammation in the hopes that the drugs she has prescribed will cool the red-hot coal down to the point where it is no longer generating the dead scar tissue known as cirrhosis. It is the cirrhosis that is life threatening because it interferes with blood circulation and prevents your liver from doing the important work that only it can perform.

Occasionally, that red-hot coal will flame up and start an uncontrollable raging fire inside your liver. If that happens—and it is rare—you will need a transplant immediately. However, most of the time your doctor will see the need for a transplant coming well in advance, often as far away as two years or more. Your doctor's estimate of when you will need a transplant will be based on how well you respond to treatment for the major complications that arise—bleeding varices and ascites.

Patient evaluation

Long before you need a transplant, your doctor will send you to the transplant center you have agreed upon so that you can undergo an evaluation to determine if you are a candidate for a liver transplant. In most instances, you will be interviewed and evaluated by a transplant surgeon, a hepatologist, a psychiatrist, and a social worker. If you have any special health needs, you may also be evaluated by a cardiologist (heart doctor), pulmonologist (lung doctor), or other specialist.

If the interviews and examinations indicate that you are a candidate for a transplant, you may then be asked to undergo a series of tests, such as an MRI or an ultrasound (to gather images of your liver); an echocardiogram and a stress test for your heart; a chest X-ray; a colonoscopy if you are over fifty years old; an endoscopic exam to see if you have esophageal varices; a dental evaluation; and additional blood tests.

If the tests indicate that you are a good candidate for a transplant, you will be interviewed by a financial officer at the center to determine if you have the money to pay for a transplant. Costs vary from center to center, but, generally speaking, your surgery and postoperative care will cost $100,000 to $200,000. If you have insurance, the financial officer will want to confirm that your coverage includes a liver transplant. If it does, then you will be asked how you will pay for the costs not covered by your policy. If you do not have insurance—and the percentage of Americans who do not is now around a staggering 40 percent—the center will determine if you qualify for one of various assistance programs.

If you are accepted by the transplant center, your name will be added to the national waiting list. The changes that the Department of Health and Human Services made in the national organ transplant procedure as a result of the Mantle and Hagman surgeries means that organs are now allocated on the basis of medical urgency, not the time you spend on the waiting list. The level of your "urgency" will be measured by what is called a

MELD score (Model for End-stage Liver Disease). Basically, it is a formula for determining the likelihood of your death within three months. The formula is **3.8 x log (e) (bilirubin mg/dl) + 11.2 x log (e) (INR) + 9.6 log (e) (creatinine mg/dl)**.

Don't be intimidated by the formula. There are numerous Web sites that help you determine your own MELD score. All you need are your test results for bilirubin, INR, and creatinine. Scores range from 6 to 40, with a score of 40 representing the sickest patient.

The most important thing you need to remember about the evaluation process is that you should not undertake it alone. Take someone with you, a family member or a close friend, to the evaluation so that you will have a separate set of eyes and ears and someone to accompany you through what most people find to be a stressful and tiring experience. You will be flooded with information and you will need someone with you to help you remember what was said.

Under what circumstances could you be rejected?

There is no constitutional right to a liver transplant. The medical profession has established a set of standards based on the probability of success. You will likely be turned down for a liver transplant if you answer yes to any of the following questions:

○ Do you drink alcohol or use heroin?
○ Do you have AIDS?
○ Do you have cancer in an organ other than the liver?
○ Do you have a severe infection?
○ Do you have advanced heart or lung disease?
○ If your cirrhosis was caused by alcoholic liver disease, have you had a drink during the past six months?
○ Do you have irreversible brain dysfunction?

There are other factors that would not necessarily prevent you from getting a transplant but would diminish your chances somewhat:

○ If you are sixty-five or older
○ If you are obese

○ If you have a poor psychological assessment
○ If you are without social support
○ If you have undergone prior shunts in your portal vein

What about living donors?

Living donors are an option for many patients. This usually happens when a relative or a friend offers part of his or her liver for the surgery. The first requirement is that the living donor have a blood type that is compatible with that of the patient. Otherwise the living donor must meet the same requirements as the patient and undergo a similar evaluation.

Complications for the donor are rare, but they must be weighed by the donor against the possible benefits for the patient. The success rate for this type of surgery is comparable to that of a conventional transplant. Since 1989, when the first living-donor transplant was performed, more than 2,000 living-donor surgeries have taken place.

Liver donors can expect a hospital stay of less than one week, but it can take a month or more for the donor to feel strong enough to return to work. Within a year's time, that portion of the donor's liver that was removed will have completely grown back.

Surgery

When a liver becomes available for you, you will be called and asked to report to the hospital. You should already have your bags packed so that you will be able to get to the hospital as quickly as possible.

You will be examined to make certain that nothing has occurred in your body to make surgery inadvisable, and then you will be prepped for the operation. That procedure usually begins with a nurse taking your temperature, pulse, and blood pressure. After that, an IV line will be attached to your arm and blood will be drawn and sent to the laboratory. You may also undergo a chest X-ray and an EKG. Before you are taken to the operating room, your abdomen and arms will be scrubbed with an antibacterial solution and you may be given a sedative to help you relax. Once you arrive in the operating room, additional IV lines will be attached and you will be given anesthesia.

All of that usually happens fairly quickly, since the doctors don't want to keep your new liver on ice for very long! You were one of 18,000 people on the waiting list and one of only 4,000 people each year to receive a liver. Count your blessings.

Removing your old liver is not time consuming. It is cut away from its attachments, examined for possible tumors, and put aside. Attaching your new liver *is* time consuming and requires great surgical skill, primarily because of the numerous blood vessels that must be joined with your new liver. As a result, bleeding is the biggest complication that your surgeon will face. You may suffer massive blood loss and require many units of plasma, red blood cells, and platelets. The most complicated part of the surgery is the attachment of the bile duct from the new liver to the tissue that remains in place where your old liver was removed.

When you awaken from surgery, you will be in the surgical ICU. You may be on a respirator and you may discover that you have been connected to a kidney dialysis machine. Your doctors' biggest concern will be whether your body will reject your new liver. They will make that determination by examining your blood for bilirubin, ALT, and AST levels.

Complications

Complications can occur at any time after the surgery. If the complications are due to rejection, your doctor will monitor it through your blood work and prescribe appropriate medications to control the rejection. Your bilirubin, AST, and ALT levels will be watched with great care, since they are a good measurement of how well your new liver is adjusting to your body.

If the complications are due to bile leakage, it may be possible to correct them with endoscopic techniques. If the complications are due to bleeding—and this is the most common complication—surgery may be necessary to stop it. After your initial surgery, you should prepare yourself emotionally for a return trip to the operating room, since it is so common.

This is when it is essential for you to maintain a positive attitude. Any complications have the potential to be serious, but you should remind yourself that your doctors expect complications and they have the expertise to deal with them.

Dealing with anxiety

One of the most common symptoms experienced by patients before and after undergoing a transplant is anxiety. A liver transplant offers life to people with end-stage liver disease, but it is a life that can be stressful if it is not well managed.

Before the transplant, patients must live with the stress of dealing with complications such as bleeding varices, ascites, and encephalopathy. Also, adding to the anxiety level is the financial cost of the transplant.

Once the surgery is over, the patient experiences a sense of relief as the problems associated with the complications disappear, only to soon be overcome by a new set of anxieties. Financial stress remains a cause of anxiety, since the drugs that must be taken for the remainder of the patient's life average about $10,000 a year; but the main stressors are the life-threatening complications associated with organ rejection and infection.

A 1997 study conducted at Baylor University Medical Center in Dallas, Texas, found that a patient's failure to cope with the anxiety of transplant surgery can affect the length of hospital stay and the occurrence of complications such as rejection and infection. Susan M. Chappell, author of the study, wrote that the emotional support of nurses was critical to the management of the patient's anxiety.

If your odds of avoiding organ rejection and infection are increased by minimizing your anxiety level, as this study indicates, I think it would be to your benefit to have a relationship with a social worker or a therapist prior to the surgery, so that you can work on the sources of your anxiety. I also think it would be beneficial for you to ask your therapist to work with you in the hospital during recovery, even to the point of sitting in on your discussions with your doctors so that the therapist can explain things to you that you may have missed.

Life after the transplant

If all goes well, you will leave the hospital less than two weeks after your surgery. You will probably be asked to return once a week for evaluation. The frequency of your visits will be cut back as your health stabilizes.

The main focus of your doctors at that point will be organ rejection and infection. The challenge for your doctors is to balance your medications. You must be given enough prednisone to suppress your immune system, so that your body will not attack your new liver, but not so much that it will open the door to a life-threatening infection.

Once you pass the hurdles associated with bleeding, organ rejection, and infection, your doctors will be concerned that whatever caused your cirrhosis does not return to damage your new liver. If your disease was caused by alcohol and you do not drink following surgery, your cirrhosis will not return. If your disease was caused by hepatitis B or C, you are at risk for reinfection. Patients at least risk for reoccurrence of cirrhosis following a transplant are those diagnosed with autoimmune hepatitis, primary biliary cirrhosis, and **primary sclerosing cholangitis**.

The five-year survival rate varies from hospital to hospital, but the average is in the 80 to 90 percent range. Once you have had your surgery and bypassed the mileposts for various complications, you can look forward to a normal life expectancy, although you will have to take medications for the rest of your life. The drugs are expensive, but they are very effective, and if you take them as prescribed, your odds of needing additional medical treatment for problems related to cirrhosis or transplant surgery are slim.

IN A SENTENCE:

> *A liver transplant offers new life to those with end-stage liver disease.*

You Always Have Choices

NOW THAT you have been living with cirrhosis for a year, you realize that one of the most striking characteristics of the disease is the opportunity it affords you to make choices in your life. You understand that your prognosis, to a great extent, depends on the choices you make about your lifestyle and treatment options.

Unless you have a rare acute condition, you understand that you have time to do many of the things that you have been postponing for so many years. I am not going to tell you that having cirrhosis is a blessing, for that is obviously not the case; but I will say that it provides you with the opportunity to more fully explore life's blessings.

Growing up in Little Rock in the 1960s, Robert Palmer played saxophone and clarinet in a series of blues, rock, and jazz bands, but it wasn't in the cards for Palmer to make his mark as a musician. So he did the next best thing—he became a music journalist, and in 1976 became the first pop music writer for the *New York Times*, eventually becoming the country's premier rock critic.

In 1985, Palmer was diagnosed with a severe case of hepatitis. At that time there were only three categories of hepatitis—hepatitis A, the virus of which was discovered in 1973, hepatitis B, the virus of which was identified in 1963, and a broad category called non-A-non-B hepatitis (which meant that it was neither A nor B). Palmer's illness fell in the latter category, though he subsequently learned that he had hepatitis C.

The same year that he was diagnosed with hepatitis, he published a biography of the Rolling Stones. Palmer's hepatitis appeared to resolve itself, and he continued with a busy schedule, but three years later it flared up again, prompting him to resign from his position at the *New York Times*. He moved to north Mississippi with his wife, JoBeth, and immersed himself in his passion for music more than ever before.

Palmer decided his hepatitis and liver disease were not going to get in the way of his continuing to live his dreams. He reveled in his new freelance lifestyle, writing and codirecting the documentary *The World According to John Coltrane*, producing albums for R. L. Burnside, Junior Kimbrough, and Cedell Davis, and serving as a consultant to a highly acclaimed ten-hour television miniseries, *Rock & Roll*, which was produced by WGBH in Boston. Unfortunately, his hepatitis flared up once again, more virulent than the previous episodes. In need of treatment, he was turned away from several hospitals because he no longer had health insurance.

In August 1996, he was admitted to Little Rock's University of Arkansas Medical Center in critical condition with kidney failure and liver failure due to cirrhosis. Doctors were able to stabilize his condition so that he could be transferred to Westchester County Medical Center in New York, where he was put on the waiting list for a liver transplant.

A number of recording artists, including Bonnie Raitt, Sonic Youth, and Alex Chilton, organized concerts in several cities to raise money for his transplant, which was estimated to cost about $100,000. Sadly, a liver was not immediately available and he died two months after arriving at the hospital, listening to his favorite music with his wife at his side. He was one of 954 people in the United States who died that year waiting for a liver transplant.

There is no "best" way to proceed

When people learn they have cirrhosis, they typically take one of two attitudes—they either withdraw from others and isolate themselves, fearful of any change in their life, or they take Palmer's approach and rearrange their life in an effort to reach out for new experiences.

For some people, withdrawal allows them to get in touch with their own feelings. In such a situation, introspection can take on some of the qualities of a powerful narcotic. For others, new experiences seem like a better investment of their time. Palmer looked at his life the way it was and considered what it could be if he pursued some of his dreams, and he chose the latter.

Would he have been better off if he had kept his newspaper job—and his health insurance—and rolled the dice in favor of a longer life? He might be alive today if that had been his choice, but he obviously decided that a life of sameness was not what he wanted. There were things that he wanted to accomplish, even if it meant risking a shorter life. Becoming a record producer had been one of his goals—and he realized that ambition, producing a number of artists on the Fat Possum blues label. The price he paid for that experience was less time. Who's to say he was right or wrong?

Learning that you have cirrhosis forces you to make decisions that you probably never thought you would have to make. There is no universal "right" decision, because each of us is different. But living with this condition can also open you up to positive experiences that you never would have otherwise.

What Edith K. remembers most about the day she learned that she had cirrhosis was the snowstorm that dropped six inches of snow on the streets. Simply getting to the doctor's office that day was a struggle. During the fifteen minutes that she sat alone in the examining room, she looked out the window as the snow swirled and cascaded onto passersby on the sidewalks below. She felt lucky to be in a warm, dry room.

Years later, when she looked back on that day, she marveled that she didn't remember much about her drive home. It was all a blur in her memory. For the next couple of weeks, time stopped still as she considered her options. She had never married and she had no children. The question she kept asking herself was, "What do I do next?"

At age forty-five, she figured that she was midway through her life (her mother had lived to ninety-two). She loved her job—she taught art at a community college—but she questioned whether she wanted to remain in that position until retirement. She was single and had no strong attachments to anyone. Her lifelong dream had been to travel to South America to study the region's art.

As the days went by after her diagnosis, she found herself thinking more and more about her dreams. One year, to the day, after her diagnosis, she closed the door to her apartment and boarded a plane to Peru. As it turned out, it was the right choice for her. She thrived on Peruvian culture and made a new life for herself as a college art instructor. The medical care she received was superb, and the new friendships she made opened new areas of understanding for her. She lived another forty years and never once looked back.

Choices—they are there for the taking.

IN A SENTENCE:

You are the only person who can decide what is best for you.

learning

Winning Your Battle with Cirrhosis

BY THE end of the first year, you will know if you are a winner. By that I don't mean whether or not you have developed complications of cirrhosis, or received a liver transplant, but whether you have developed a lifesaving attitude toward your disease.

Cirrhosis is a disease that demands a lot from its patients. It is important that you follow your doctor's treatment instructions and take your medication, but it takes more than that to prevail over such a stubborn disease. It takes positive thinking.

In most instances, cirrhosis patients have control over their destiny.

Medicine has changed over the past five or six years. In years past, doctors made a diagnosis and then decided on your treatment. Today, your doctor is more likely to offer you several treatments, without stating his or her preference. Instead, you will be asked to read up all you can on the various treatments and then decide for yourself. This is especially true with a disease like cirrhosis, in which treatment is more of an art than a science.

Be positive

A 2001 study conducted by Johns Hopkins Center for Health Promotion found that a positive outlook offered the strongest known protection for adults at risk for heart disease. According to the study, people with a good attitude were only half as likely as their less optimistic counterparts of experiencing a heart attack.

The study focused on 586 adults aged thirty to fifty-nine with no symptoms of heart disease but whose brothers and sisters had been diagnosed with early heart disease. Diane M. Becker, author of the study, concluded that people with a positive attitude produce lower levels of stress hormones that help protect them from disease. Other studies have reported that people with a positive attitude may delay the aging process and that physical performance can be influenced by a positive attitude.

Speaking as a social worker, there is no doubt in my mind that a positive attitude can affect the progress of your cirrhosis. It can bolster your immune system and it can reduce the output of stress-related hormones and enzymes that burden your liver cells.

Do you have a positive or negative attitude?

Positive Attitude	Negative Attitude
You usually expect the best.	You usually expect the worst.
You look on the bright side of life.	You look on the dark side of life.
You aren't surprised if things go. your way.	You hardly ever expect things to go your way.
You have an easy time praising others.	You have a difficult time praising others.

If you are the person in the Positive Attitude column, there's not much anyone needs to do to motivate you about your approach to treating your cirrhosis. You have an advantage going into treatment. However, if you are the person in the Negative Attitude column, you are at a disadvantage. It is not easy to change negative thinking. It has probably been with you for most of your life. Having said that, the positive-attitude person inside me insists that you can do it if you try.

If you have a hard time intellectualizing the concept of changing your attitude, I suggest you approach it from a more emotional level. Read inspirational stories. Watch inspirational movies. A good fiction writer or a good moviemaker has the ability to make you *feel* the inspirational message in their art. For the short term, create a new world order for your life. Stop reading newspapers or watching television news, where you are likely to be exposed to war, disease, and famine, and create your own inspirational world.

Your problem is that you don't know what it feels like to have a positive attitude. Once you have inundated yourself with inspirational books and movies, you will understand that feeling a little better. At that point, you need to start displaying positive behavior. Compliment your friends and coworkers on how they look. Join a community organization that helps the needy. Become a doer of positive things.

Whether you have a positive or a negative attitude, it is essential that you maintain your personal appearance. It is easy to fall into the trap of justifying lapses in good grooming by blaming it on your cirrhosis. You've got to fight that urge. It is essential that you shower or bathe every day, whether you have anyplace to go or not. It is important that you keep your regular appointments at the barber shop or beauty salon. Instead of wearing the same clothes for several days in a row, purchase new clothes that will tell the world that you are optimistic about your future.

Be healthy

Aside from positive thinking, the most important things you can do to improve your prognosis are (1) adopt a healthy lifestyle in which you exercise every day, even if it is only a thirty-minute walk, and (2) follow a diet that is calculated to provide you with maximum nourishment. Cirrhosis is not a disease that has a miracle cure that can be administered by a machine or a pill. It can only be beaten by hard work.

Be strong

By being strong, I mean that you should stand tall and fight the urge to isolate yourself from friends and loved ones. Giving up is the easy way out. It's not difficult to find excuses not to do things with family and friends. You can blame it on your cirrhosis. In fact, there is something seductive about isolation. It beckons with a knowing nod and promises you peace of mind. If you listen, your life will be history before you know it.

It takes strength to maintain relationships with friends, family, and co-workers when you know that you have a disease that they do not have. It takes strength to stay in the room with them when they talk about their retirement plans or the vacation homes they are going to build for their old age. It takes strength to listen to the petty relationship, shopping, or grooming "problems" they have, when all you really want to do is shout at the top of your voice, "I'm dying here, you know!"

Be strong by staying in life's game. It hasn't beaten you yet, and it may not beat you for many years to come, if ever. As you know by now, many cirrhosis patients die of something else.

Keep learning

The fact that you are reading this book is an indication that you understand the importance of learning all that you can about cirrhosis. It is essential that you keep reading everything you can. Scientific knowledge about this disease increases each day, and it is important that you update yourself about new discoveries. The more you know about cirrhosis, the more effective you can be at surviving it.

I am confident that researchers will find a cure for this disease. Meanwhile, my best wishes go to you and your loved ones—indeed, to anyone who has cirrhosis.

IN A SENTENCE:

> *You have the power to be a winner.*

Glossary

ACUPUNCTURE: A tool of traditional Chinese medicine, acupuncture is the insertion of very small needles into the skin at sites called acupuncture points. Its purpose is to change the "energy flow" of the body.

AFLATOXIN: A fungus that grows in foods such as peanuts, soybeans, corn and rice in hot, humid conditions for long periods of time. It is one of the most powerful known carcinogens.

ALANINE AMINOTRANSFERASE (ALT OR SGPT): A liver enzyme that is measured in routine laboratory tests. When included with a second enzyme, aspartate aminotransferase, the two are referred to as transaminases.

ALBUMIN: A protein produced by the liver.

ALKALINE PHOSPHATASE (AP): A liver enzyme that is usually grouped together with gamma-glutamyl transferase (GGTP) and identified as cholestatic liver enzymes. Elevation is usually an indication of bile duct disease.

ALPHA 1-ANTITRYPSIN: A liver enzyme that protects tissue from enzymes from inflammatory cells, especially elastase. Alpha 1-antitrypsin deficiency is a hereditary disorder that causes tissue breakdowns that can lead to liver cirrhosis.

ASCITES: The fluid that accumulates in the abdominal cavity as a result of cirrhosis.

ASPARTATE AMINOTRANSFERASE (AST OR SGOT): A liver enzyme that is measured in routine laboratory tests. When included with a second enzyme, alanine aminotransferase, the two are referred to as transaminases.

AUTOIMMUNE HEPATITIS: An uncommon chronic liver disease that can lead to cirrhosis. It is liver inflammation that is caused by a person's immune system attacking the liver. It can occur in men or women, but it mostly affects women. The cause of autoimmune hepatitis is not known. It is not associated with the viruses that cause hepatitis.

AZATHIOPRINE: A steroid-sparing drug that allows a patient to be treated with lower doses of prednisone. It is also used as an antirejection drug for kidney transplants.

BAYTRIL: A veterinary antibiotic that is given to poultry to combat infection. It is the equivalent of Cipro, a drug known to cause liver damage.

BILIRUBIN: A greenish-yellow substance made from chemically converted hemoglobin. It is a good indicator of a liver's efficiency. Damaged livers accumulate bilirubin in the blood, a process that turns the skin yellow and the urine dark-yellow or brown.

CAROTENOIDS: Fat-soluble pigments found in plants that are characteristically bright red, orange, or yellow. They serve as antioxidants and they are often a source of vitamin A.

CHILD-PUGH: A rating scale that allows doctors to determine the different stages of cirrhotic development.

CIPRO (CIPROFLOXACIN): A fluorinated antibiotic that is used to treat a wide range of infections. It is known to cause liver failure.

CRYPTOGENIC CIRRHOSIS: Cirrhosis for which there is no known cause.

ENCEPHALOPATHY: A brain dysfunction caused by the accumulation of toxic chemicals in the blood. This occurs in cirrhosis when the liver is unable to remove toxic chemicals, the most easily identified being ammonia.

EDEMA: Swelling of the legs due to complications of cirrhosis.

ESOPHAGEAL VARICES: Enlarged veins in the esophagus similar to varicose veins. They develop when cirrhosis blocks blood from flowing through the liver. If the veins rupture, it can lead to life-threatening bleeding.

FETAL ALCOHOL SYNDROME: A condition characterized by abnormal facial features, nervous system problems, and growth retardation. It can occur if a woman drinks alcohol during her pregnancy. Children with FAS typically have learning and behavioral problems.

GALACTOSEMIA: A disorder that affects how the body processes sugars such as galactose. If not treated, it can lead to liver dysfunction.

GAMMA-GLUTAMYL TRANSFERASE (GGTP): A liver enzyme measured on routine liver function tests.

GASTRIC VARICES: Enlarged veins in the stomach similar to varicose veins. If they rupture, it can lead to life-threatening bleeding.

GLYCOGEN STORAGE DISEASE: One of several metabolism disorders that result from enzyme defects that affect the processing of glycogen.

GYNECOMASTIA: An enlargement of the male breast caused by faulty estrogen production in the liver.

HEMOCHROMATOSIS: A condition that causes iron to accumulate in the liver.

HEPATIC ARTERY: The artery that enters the liver from the aorta, which carries blood from the heart.

HEPATITIS A: An inflammation of the liver due to a virus called hepatitis A. Once known as "infectious hepatitis," it is very contagious, but it does not progress to a chronic condition, nor does it lead to cirrhosis. Food is a common transmission vehicle for the disease; it is associated with restaurant food.

HEPATITIS B: An inflammation of the liver due to a virus called hepatitis B. Once known as "serum hepatitis," it is the single greatest cause of cirrhosis and liver cancer worldwide—but not in the United States. It is commonly transmitted through blood, semen, vaginal secretions, and, possibly, saliva.

HEPATITIS C: An inflammation of the liver due to a virus called hepatitis C. It is the most common cause of cirrhosis and liver cancer in the United States. It can be transmitted by blood-to-blood contact (blood transfusions), intravenous drug use, tattooing and body piercing, and sexual contact—and it can be transmitted from mother to child.

HEPATITIS D: An inflammation of the liver due to a virus called hepatitis delta (HDV). It is unique in that it can only live in people who already have hepatitis B. It is transmitted through blood or sexual contact, or from mother to child.

HEPATITIS E: An inflammation of the liver due to a virus in the calicivirus category. It is an acute infection that does not develop into a chronic condition. Thus far, the disease does not occur in the United States. Americans who have the disease picked it up traveling outside the country. Contaminated water is the most common means of transmission.

HEPATOCELLULAR CARCINOMA: Cancer of the liver.

HEPATOCYTES: The chief functional cells of the liver. They perform an astonishing workload and account for 80 percent of the liver's mass.

INTERFERON: An antiviral drug that is effective in treating people with hepatitis B and C. The drug has also proven effective in fighting cancer and in regulating the immune system.

JAUNDICE: A condition in which the skin and the whites of the eyes become yellow due to a faulty processing of bilirubin. Associated with hepatitis A and B, it can occur in association with acute liver failure due to cirrhosis.

KASAI PROCEDURE: An operation performed on children in which damaged bile ducts are replaced with a piece of the infant's intestine.

LIVER ENZYMES: Proteins that promote specific chemical reactions within the liver.

LUPUS: An autoimmune disease that can affect any system in the body.

METABOLIZE: The process through which the liver breaks down chemicals into various elements so that they can be used by the body.

MILK THISTLE (SILYMARIN): The most widely used herb for the treatment of liver disease. In use for hundreds of years, herbalists claim that it is an effective treatment for cirrhosis. Medical doctors are reluctant to prescribe it, but most say that it is safe.

NONALCOHOLIC FATTY LIVER DISEASE (NAFLD): The most common liver disease in the United States. It is called "nonalcoholic" because the biopsies of people with this disease are almost identical to those of people with alcoholic liver disease. Despite the similarities, NAFLD is considered a reversible condition. Nonalcoholic steatohepatitis (NASH) is the name of fatty liver disease that has progressed to inflammation or cirrhosis.

OZONE THERAPY: A form of therapy that attacks viruses by increasing their exposure to oxygen.

PERCUTANEOUS BIOPSY: When the skin is penetrated for the purpose of gathering tissue samples for examination by a pathologist.

PORTAL VEIN: Despite its name, the portal vein carries blood into the liver, most notably from the pancreas, spleen, and small intestines.

PREDNISONE: A synthetic hormone that is similar to the steroids produced naturally by the body. It is the preferred drug for the treatment of autoimmune hepatitis. It is also used for transplant patients.

PRIMARY HEPATOCELLULAR CARCINOMA: A cancer that originates in the liver. It is the most common primary liver cancer in the world, and the most common cancer linked to hepatitis C.

PRIMARY SCLEROSING CHOLANGITIS: A liver disease caused by an autoimmune disorder. If the disease progresses to cirrhosis, a liver transplant may be needed. Treatment focuses on slowing the disease's progression and managing symptoms.

RETINOIDS: Natural or synthetic versions of vitamin A that are used in chemotherapy.

RUBBER BAND LITIGATION: Also known as sclerotherapy, it is performed by placing a rubber band on the varices for the purpose of stopping bleeding. It works by creating a blood clot within the vein.

SCLEROTHERAPY: A process by which small varicose veins are injected with a concentrated salt or medicated solutions. It is used to stop bleeding from varices in the esophagus and the stomach.

SINUSOIDS: Specialized capillaries in the liver.

SPLENOMEGALY: Enlargement of the spleen. It occurs in cirrhosis patients when blood backs up into the spleen because of elevated pressure in the liver.

SPONTANEOUS PERITONITIS SCLEROTHERAPY: The injection of a chemical solution into the varicose vein made visible by the endoscope.

TRANSAMINASES (AST AND ALT): The two liver enzymes known as aspartate aminotransferase and alanine aminotransferase.

WILSON'S DISEASE: A genetic disorder that is usually fatal unless detected early. It is transmitted through recessive genes, which means it is not gender exclusive. Two abnormal genes must be present for the disease to develop.

Resources

Books

Bruce, Cara, and Lisa Montanarelli. *Hepatitis C: The First Year*. New York: Marlowe & Co., 2002.

Chopra, Sanjiv. *Dr. Sanjiv Chopra's Liver Book*. New York: Pocket Books, 2001.

Cohen, Jay S. *Over Dose: Prescription Drugs, Side Effects and Your Health*. New York: Jeremy P. Tarcher/Putnam, 2004.

Hobbs, Christopher. *Natural Therapy for Your Liver*. New York: Avery, 2002.

Kidman, Antony. *From Thought to Action*. St. Leonards, Australia: Biochemical & General Services, 1988.

Laskow, Leonard. *Healing with Love*. New York: Harper San Francisco, 1992.

MacNutt, Father Francis. *Healing*. New York: Bantam Books, 1977.

Moody Jr., Raymond A. *Life after Life*. New York: Bantam Books, 1976.

Palmer, Melissa. *Dr. Melissa Palmer's Guide to Hepatitis and Liver Disease*. New York: Avery, 2004.

Scheinberg, I. H. "Wilson's Disease." In: *Harrison's Principles of Internal Medicine*. New York: McGraw-Hill, 1994.

Shomon, Mary J. *Living Well with Autoimmune Disease*. New York: HarperCollins, 2002.

Siegel, Bernie S. *Love, Medicine & Miracles*. New York: Harper & Row Publishers, 1986.

Worman, Howard J. *The Liver Disorders Sourcebook*. Chicago: Lowell House, 1999.

Zukerman, Eugenia, and Julie R. Ingelfinger. *Coping with Prednisone*. New York: St. Martin's Griffin, 1997.

Periodicals

Associated Press. "Report Finds Wide Disparity in Survival in Heart, Liver Transplants." October 13, 1999.

Bhatti, Ahsan M., and Thomas R. Riley. "Preventive Strategies in Chronic Liver Disease: Part II: Cirrhosis." *American Family Physician*, November 15, 2001.

Basto, Samanta Teixeira, and Bernardo Haddock Lobo Goulart. "Wilson's Disease." *medstudents.com*.

Carey, Benedict. "Long-Awaited Medical Study Questions the Power of Prayer." *The New York Times*, March 31, 2006.

Chappell, Susan M. "Anxiety in Liver Transplant Patients." *MedSurg Nursing*, April 1, 1997.

Cowan, Rachel. "Healing the Soul, Healing the World." *Nathan Cummings Foundation Annual Report*, 1995.

DeAngelis, Tori. "What's to Blame for the Surge in Super-size Americans?" *Monitor on Psychology*, January 2004.

Estrada, Benjamin. "Treatment of Hepatitis B in Children." *Infections in Medicine*, 16(2): 79, 1999. Accessed at www.medscape.com.

Harris, Gardiner. "Drug Safety System Is Broken." *The New York Times*, June 9, 2005.

Hicks, Doris. "Consumers: Know the Facts about Eating Raw Shellfish." *MAS Note: University of Delaware Sea Grant Marine Advisory Service*, February 1995.

Laland, Stephanie. "The Healing Power of Love—A True Story," adapted from *Animal Angels*. New York: Conari Press, 2005.

Lillis, Rebecca A., et al. "A Fish Hook and Liver Disease: Revisiting an Old Enemy." *Journal of the Louisiana State Medical Society*, January/February 2002.

Mihas, Anastasios A. "Cirrhosis of the Liver." *Postgraduate Medicine* 109:2, February 2001.

Newton, Julia L., et al. "Presentation and Mortality of Primary Biliary Cirrhosis in Older Patients." *Age and Ageing*, 2000.

Sered, Susan Starr. "Healing and Religion: A Jewish Perspective." *Yale Journal for Humanities in Medicine*, January 28, 2002.

Sellner, H. Ascher. "What You Should Know about Wilson's Disease." Wilson's Disease Association, 1997, accessed at: www.wilsonsdisease.org.

Williams, Martin. "The Healing Power of Pets." *Reader's Digest*, August 2000.

General Sources of Information

2005 OPTN/SRTR Annual Report (www.ustransplant.org)

American Cancer Society (www.cancer.org)

American Liver Foundation (www.liverfoundation.org)

Cincinnati Children's Hospital (www.cincinnatichildrens.org)

WNBC, New York, NY. "Diet and Cirrhosis: What Should You Be Eating?" Interview with Dr. Carol Semrad, Presbyterian Hospital, and Dr. Howard J. Worman, Presbyterian Hospital.

Mayo Clinic (www.mayoclinic.com)

National Institute of Mental Health (www.nimh.nih.gov)

National Center for Health Statistics (www.cdc.gov/nchs)

U.S. Centers for Disease Control and Prevention (www.cdc.gov)

U.S. Food and Drug Administration (www.fda.gov)

United Network for Organ Sharing (www.unos.org)

The Merck Manual of Diagnosis and Therapy (www.merck.com)

Tulane University Center for Abdominal Transplant (www.tulanetransplant.com)

University of Southern California Department of Surgery (www.surgery.usc.edu)

Acknowledgments

I would like to thank my editor, Katie McHugh; the acquiring editor, Sue McCloskey; Fredric Regenstein, MD, and Charles Hall, MD, for taking such good care of me and educating me on the nuances of cirrhosis; Elizabeth Mitchell, MD, for protecting my eyesight; Kim Warren-Ellis, MD; Jim Richardson; my sister, Susan McCaskill; my mother, Juanita Caldwell; Billy Watkins and Marshall Ramsey, for offering me encouragement; my good friend Alex Alston; and, during the writing process, Allie and Mattie, two award-worthy cocker spaniels, for not barking when the squirrels in the backyard tormented them with their antics.

Index

A

abalation procedures, 166
acetaminophen, 33–34, 56, 64,
    124–25
acetysalicylic acid, 65
acupuncture, 195–96
acute hepatitis, 47, 50
addictions, 90–95, 196. *See also*
    alcohol
additives in foods, 44–45
advance directives, 112–13
aflatoxin, 163–64
AFP (alpha-fetoprotein), 29, 85,
    164–65
age-related sleep issues, 160
albumin
    low level of, 16–17, 28–29, 84,
        139–41, 147
    overview, 6, 87–88
alcohol
    abusing, 6, 33, 37, 120
    and acetaminophen, 56
    eliminating, 11–12, 92–93
    liver's metabolism of, 97–98
    and loss of libido, 202
    and recreational drugs, 12, 33,
        90–95, 125, 164, 218–19
    withdrawal, 120
alcoholic cirrhosis, 96–99, 120, 162,
    163
alcoholic fatty liver, 98
alcoholic hepatitis, 82, 83, 98

Alcoholics Anonymous, 92–93, 104
alpha 1-antitrypsin deficiency, 162,
    170
ALT (alanine aminotransferase),
    27–28, 64, 73, 82–83, 122, 233
alternative treatments, 193–99, 209,
    220
Americans with Disabilities Act, 39,
    181–82
ammonia, 17–18
anabolic steroids, 66, 164
anal intercourse, 13, 49
anemia, 153
anesthetics, adverse reactions to, 63
antibiotics, 33, 34, 59, 147, 150
antidiscrimination laws, 39, 181–83
antifibrotics, 222
anti-LKM antibodies, 73
AP (alkaline phosphatase), 27–28, 73,
    83
ascites
    overview, 8, 17, 87–88, 139–40
    and salt in diet, 44–45, 147
    and SSI benefits, 111
    treatment options, 147–48
aspirin, 65
AST (aspartate aminotransferase),
    27–28, 64, 73, 82–83, 122, 233
attitude adjustments, 11–14, 167,
    191–92, 208, 240–43
autoimmune disorder (PBC),
    125–26

autoimmune hepatitis, 6, 71–75, 122–23,
    162, 170, 209
azathioprine, 74, 122–23, 170

B

Bethea, Charles, 189
bilary atresia, 170–71
bile, 16
bilirubin
    after liver transplant, 233
    elevated levels, 28, 73, 83, 111, 231
    overview, 6, 16, 87–88
    and SSI benefits, 111
biotin, 58
bleeding varices, 111, 126, 133, 143–44,
    149–50, 230
blood, transmission through, 50
blood clotting, 17, 56, 65, 74
blood pressure medications, 66, 72
blood tests, 27–29, 81–82. *See also specific
    tests*
body mass index (BMI), 135
breasts
    atrophy, 19, 200, 202–3
    enlargement, 18–19, 141–42, 148
Busuttil, Ronald, 227

C

calcium supplements, 60–61
carotenoids, 56
cataracts, 142–43
Chappell, Susan M., 234
Child-Pugh score, 87–89
children, 39, 49, 50
children with cirrhosis, 168–72
chlorambucil, 126
cholesterol, 18, 66, 131
Chopra, Sanjiv, 65, 75, 120, 121, 126
chronic hepatitis, 47–48, 50
cigarette smoking, 12, 163
circadian rhythm disorders, 159–60
cirrhosis, 6–8, 32–34, 40–41, 99, 218–22.
    See also specific types of cirrhosis
clinical trials, 109, 209, 221
colchicine, 126
comfrey, 127
complete blood count (CBC), 28
complications
    bleeding varices, 111, 126, 133, 143–44,
        149–50, 230
    decrease in drug metabolism, 142
    edema, 8, 17, 140–41, 147–48
    enlarged liver and spleen, 141–42, 148
    glaucoma and cataracts, 142–43, 148
    gynecomastia, 18–19, 141–42, 148
    from immune system suppression, 74–75,
        221, 234–35
    osteoporosis, 60–61, 132–33, 143, 149

overview, 89, 139–40, 146
    of transplant, 221, 233
    See also ascites; encephalopathy
copper poisoning. *See* Wilson's disease
Coumadin, 65
Cowan, Rachel, 190–91
cryptogenic cirrhosis, 127, 176
CT or CAT scan, 30–31, 86, 164–65
cyanocobalamin, 58
cyclosporine, 126
cystic fibrosis, 171

D

death, 6–7, 78, 79, 236–37
DEET-based products, 132
delta gent, 53
Denver shunt, 148
depression, 4, 91, 152–56, 179–80
detoxification, 93, 94
diabetes, medications for, 66
diagnosis
    of autoimmune hepatitis, 72–73
    emotional response to, 1–4, 115–16
    of hepatitis A, 49
    of liver cancer, 77–80, 164–65
diazepam, 65
diet, 42–46, 49, 147, 163–64, 242
dilitiazem, 66
disability insurance, 107
diuretics, 147
doctors
    and alternative therapies, 194–95, 209,
        220
    importance of honesty with, 32–33,
        175–77, 178–79
    and medication history, 62–63
    overview, 20–24, 207–10
    referral to national waiting list, 226
"do not resuscitate" order, 112–13
drug abuse treatment principles, 93–94
drug-induced liver disease, 33–34, 62–66,
    124–25, 164
drug metabolism, decrease in, 142
drugs, recreational, 12, 33, 90–95, 125, 164,
    218–19
durable power of attorney, 112–13

E

edema, 8, 17, 140–41, 147–48
Eisenberg, David, 194
emotional isolation, 137–38
emotions
    of family and friends, 69, 103
    personal response to diagnosis, 1–4,
        115–16
    as side effect or depression, 154–55
    transplant-related, 234
employers, 39–40, 181–85

encephalopathy
  from ammonia in the blood, 17–18
  and depression, 153, 155
  overview, 87–88, 140, 150, 159, 219, 234
  and protein in diet, 45, 150, 178
  and sleep disorders, 159
  and SSI benefits, 111
  treatment for, 150–51
endoscopic evaluation, 31, 87, 143, 230
endoscopic therapy, 149, 233
enflurane, 63
enlarged liver and spleen, 141–42, 148
esophageal varices, 111, 126, 133, 143–44,
  149–50, 230
estrogen, 18–19, 66
exercise, 14, 129–33, 242
expectations, patient's, 102–3
experimental treatments, 109, 209, 222

        F
family, 3, 35–39, 69, 101–3, 159, 203–5
fast food restaurants, 74–75
fatty buildup, 18
fatty liver disease, 135
fecal-to-mouth transmission, 48
fetal alcohol syndrome, 170
financial planning
  with health insurance, 106–9
  without health insurance, 109–13
fluoroquinolones, 147
folate (folic acid), 58
friends, 3, 40, 68, 103
fulminant hepatitis, 48

        G
gamma-glutamyl transferase (GGTP), 27–28,
  73, 83
gastric varices, 143
gastroenterologists, 20, 23
genetic predisposition, 34, 52, 72, 96, 125, 126
ginseng, 199
Glaser, Ronald, 68–69
glaucoma, 142–43, 148
government programs, 110–11
green tea, 199
grief, five stages of, 3
gynecomastia, 18–19, 141–42, 148

        H
Hagman, Larry, 223–24
Hall, Charles, 207–10
hallucinations, 8
halothane, 63
HDV, 53
health insurance, 106–10
Health Insurance Portability and
  Accountability Act (1996), 183
hemochromatosis, 127, 162

hepatic artery, 6
hepatic vein, 147–48
hepatitis, 47–48
hepatitis A, 48–49
hepatitis B
  in children, 169
  and liver cancer, 162
  overview, 6, 33, 49–51, 182
  transmission of, 50, 205
  treatment for, 120–21, 122
hepatitis C
  in infants, 169
  and liver cancer, 162
  overview, 6, 33, 51–53, 182, 203
  in seniors, 177–78
  transmission of, 37, 51, 205
  treatment for, 58, 121, 122
hepatitis D, 53, 121–22
hepatitis E, 53
hepatitis in children, 169
hepatitis viral serological markers test, 29, 85
hepatocellular carcinoma, 29, 161–62
hepatocytes, 15–16
herbal-related cirrhosis, 127
herbal remedies, 194, 197–99, 220
Hill, Edward, 190
HMG-CoA reductase inhibitors, 66
Hobbs, Christopher, 198
home health-care, 112

        I
ibuprofen, 33, 65
immune system, 13–14, 52, 68–69, 187–88,
  198–99, 221
immunoglobulin-A, 187
INR (international normalized ratio), 84,
  87–88, 231
insurance, 106–10
intellectual isolation, 138
interferon, 58, 120
International Autoimmune Hepatitis Scoring
  System for the Diagnosis of AIH
  guidelines, 73
international normalized ratio (INR), 84,
  87–88, 231
Internet addiction, 215–16
Internet research, 208, 212–14, 216–17
Internet support groups, 104–5, 184, 211–12
iron levels, 45–46, 55, 127
Islamic prayer tradition, 191
isolation, 70, 137–38, 156, 179–80
isoniozid (INH), 66
itching, 8, 140

        J
jaundice, 16, 49, 50, 52, 125, 140
Jewish prayer tradition, 190–91
Judd, Naomi, 199

K

Kasai procedure, 170–71
kava, 199
Kiecolt-Glaser, Janice, 68–69
Kirshnit, Carol, 187

L

lamivudine, 121
lecithin supplements, 60
LeVeen shunt, 148
licorice root, 198
life after transplants, 234–35
life expectancy estimate, 87–89
life with cirrhosis, 236–39
liver
    drug sensitivity, 63
    function estimates, 219
    purpose, 5–6, 15–19, 42, 55–56, 97–98
    tissue regeneration, 10, 169, 176
liver allocation system, 225–26
liver biopsy, 77–80
liver cancer
    causes of, 162–64
    diagnosis of, 77–80, 164–65
    overview, 29, 75, 144–45, 161–62,
        209–10
    prevention, 166–67
    treatment of, 165–66
liver enzymes
    alkaline phosphatase, 27–28, 73, 83
    ALT and AST, 27–28, 64, 73, 82–83, 122,
        233
    AP and GGTP, 27–28, 73, 83
liver-spleen scan, 30, 86–87
living donors, 232
living will, 112–13
loneliness, 70
long-term care, 111–12
love, healing through, 187–88
lupoid hepatitis, 72

M

MacNutt, Father Francis, 190
magnesium supplements, 60
Mantle, Mickey, 224
McClelland, David, 187
meat additives, 34
Medicaid, 110
medical records protections, 183–84
medical tests, 26–27, 81–82. See also specific
    tests and diseases
Medicare, 110
medications
    drug-induced liver disease from, 33–34,
        62–66, 124–25, 164
    impotence as side effect, 202
    methods for obtaining, 109–10
    sleep problems from, 158–59

for viral hepatitis, 120–22
    See also treatment options; specific
        medications
MELD score (Model for End-Stage Liver
    Disease), 230–31
memory loss, 8, 17–18
men
    breast enlargement, 18–19, 141–42, 148
    libido loss, 200, 201–2
menstruation, 13
metabolic therapies, 197
methotrexate, 65, 126
methoxyflurane, 63
microbe-carrying foods, 43–44
milk thistle, 197–98, 220
Motrin, 33, 65, 124–25
multivitamins without iron, 55, 56

N

Narcotics Anonymous, 92
national waiting list, 226, 230–31, 233
niacin, 57
nitrites or nitrates, 44
nonalcoholic fatty liver disease (NAFLD)
    biotin and, 58
NASH stage, 6, 162, 171
    and obesity, 135–36
    overview, 6, 18, 83
    treatment for, 123
nonalcoholic steatohepatitis (NASH), 6, 162,
    171

O

obesity, 46, 123, 134–38, 156, 220. See also
    diet; exercise
oral contraceptives, 65, 164
orlistat, 123
osteoporosis, 60–61, 132–33, 143, 149
ozone therapy, 196–97

P

Palmer, Melissa, 13, 59, 96, 126, 149,
    196–97
Palmer, Robert, 236–37
pantothenic acid, 57
paracentesis, 147
patient evaluation for transplant, 230–31
penicillamine, 125
percutaneous biopsy, 78
pets, healing effect of, 188
phentermine, 123
phlebotomy, 127
physical isolation, 137
physicians. See doctors
platelet count, 17, 78–79, 84–85, 141, 233
pollen as irritant, 132
portal vein, 6, 147–48
positive-action steps, 11–14

potassium, 147
poultry additives, 34
prayer, healing through, 189–91
prednisone, 74, 122–23, 129, 170, 203
pregnant women, 53–54
prescriptions. *See* medications
primary biliary cirrhosis (PBC), 125–26, 162
primary sclerosing cholangitis, 235
prothrombin, 59–60
prothrombin time (PT), 17, 28, 78–79, 84
proton pump inhibitors, 58
pyridoxine, 57

R

Rebetron, 121
Regenstein, Fredric
    on ALT/AST elevation, 64
    on cirrhosis' negative stigma, 218–19
    on cirrhotic patients, 166
    on drug-induced cirrhosis, 33
    on liver cancer and autoimmune hepatitis,
        75
    supplement recommendations, 55
    on Urso, 126
retinoids, 56
riboflavin, 57
rubber band ligation, 149

S

salad bars, 44
salt, 44–45, 147
sclerotherapy, 149
second opinions, 24–25
self-care, 67–70, 208, 240–43. *See also*
    spiritual healing
Semrad, Carol, 44–45
senior citizens with cirrhosis, 175–80
serum ceruloplasmin, 29
serum hepatitis. *See* hepatitis B
sexual activity, 12–13, 50, 200–206
sexual orientation, 32
shellfish, uncooked, 43–44
shunts, 147–48, 149–50
sibutramine, 123
Siegel, Bernie S., 188
silymarin, 197–98, 220
sinusoids, 6, 15
sleep issues, 157–60
sleep-related illnesses, 159–60
smoking, 12, 163
Social Security Disability Insurance (SSDI),
    111
social services, 110–11
social workers, 116
sonograms, 29–30, 85–86, 141, 164–65, 210
spiritual healing, 186–87
    attitude adjustments, 11–14, 167,
        191–92, 208, 240–43

living your dreams, 236–39
    self-care, 67–70, 208, 240–43
    through prayer, 189–91
spleen, enlarged, 141–42, 148
splenomegaly, 141
spontaneous peritonitis, 147
spontaneous peritonitis sclerotherapy, 31
statins, 66
stress, 13–14, 68–69, 159, 234
Supplemental Security Income (SSI), 111
support groups
    of cirrhosis patients, 103–5
    Internet-based, 104–5, 184, 211–12
    for overcoming addiction, 91–93, 104
support network, 100–101, 105
surgical removal of tumors, 165
surgical shunt, 149–50
symptoms
    breast atrophy (women), 19, 200, 202–3
    breast enlargement (men), 18–19,
        141–42, 148
    of cyanocobalamin deficiency, 58
    of depression, 153
    disease progression, 7–8, 139–40
    of folate deficiency, 58
    jaundice, 16, 49, 50, 52, 125, 140
    sleep issues, 157–60
    urine color, 16

T

tannic acid and nitrites, 44
testosterone, 66
test results, requesting a copy of, 82
tetracycline, 65, 124–25
therapy, 40, 115–18, 155–56
thiamine, 57
thymus extracts, 198–99
thyroid disorders, 153
TIPS procedure, 147–48, 150
toxin buildups, 17–18, 97, 200
transaminases, 27–28, 50–51, 64, 73, 82–83,
    122, 233
transmission of hepatitis virus, 12–13, 37, 48,
    49, 50, 51, 53, 205
transplant centers, 226–28
transplants
    anxiety related to, 234
    of celebrities, 223–24
    for children, 171
    dying while waiting for, 236–37
    life after, 234–35
    for liver cancer, 166
    living donors, 232
    preparing for, 220–21, 224–25, 229–31
    rejected patients, 231–32
    for seniors, 177–78
    the surgery, 232–33
    survival rates, 227–28

waiting list, 226, 230–31, 233
treatment options
 for autoimmune hepatitis, 74, 122–23, 170
 for bilary atresia, 170–71
 for bleeding varices, 149–50
 for edema and ascites, 147–48
 for hemochromatosis, 127
 for liver cancer, 165–66
 for NAFLD, 123
 overview, 119–20
 shunts, 147–48, 149–50
 untreatable forms of cirrhosis, 124–25, 127–28, 148
 for viral hepatitis, 120–22
 Wilson's disease, 125
 See also medications
tremors, 8
trientine, 125
triple organ transplants, 171
tumor embolization, 165–66
Tylenol, 33–34, 56, 64, 124

u

ultrasound, 29–30, 85–86, 141, 164–65, 210
United Network for Organ Sharing (UNOS), 225–26
urine color, 16
ursodiol, 123, 126

v

vacation, 68
vaccinations, 11, 122, 172
Veterans Administration, 110

Viagra, 204
vibrio vulnificus, 43
viral hepatitis, 120–22, 218–19. See also hepatitis B; hepatitis C; hepatitis D
vitamin A, 34, 56–57
vitamin A-related cirrhosis, 124
vitamin B complex, 57–58
vitamin C, 58, 123
vitamin D, 58–59
vitamin E, 59, 123
vitamin K, 17, 56, 59–60
vitamins, 34, 55–56, 61. See also specific vitamins and supplements

w

walking, 130–32
weight-bearing exercise, 132–33
weight gain, causes of, 136, 137–38
weight-loss medications, 123
Williams, Tennessee, 103–4
Wilson's disease, 29, 34, 125, 170
women
 breast atrophy, 19, 200, 202–3
 decreased interest in sex, 202–3
 and osteoporosis, 149
 period and hepatitis transmission, 13
 risk factor for cirrhosis, 97
Worman, Howard J., 72–73, 126, 169

z

zinc acetate, 125